The
CHEMISTRY
of
JOY

A Three-Step Program for Overcoming Depression
Through Western Science and Eastern Wisdom

HENRY EMMONS, M.D.
WITH RACHEL KRANZ

A FIRESIDE BOOK
Published by Simon & Schuster

New York   London   Toronto   Sydney

FIRESIDE
Rockefeller Center
1230 Avenue of the Americas
New York, NY 10020

Copyright © 2006 by Henry Emmons
All rights reserved, including the right of reproduction
in whole or in part in any form.

FIRESIDE and colophon are registered trademarks of Simon & Schuster, Inc.

For information regarding special discounts for bulk purchases,
please contact Simon & Schuster Special Sales at
1-800-456-6798 or business@simonandschuster.com

Designed by Ruth Lee-Mui

Manufactured in the United States of America

10

Library of Congress Cataloging-in-Publication Data

ISBN-13: 978-0-7432-6507-2
ISBN-10:   0-7432-6507-6

This book is dedicated to all who suffer from inner states of fear, anger, or sadness. May your reading of this work provide you with comfort and courage and give you greater skill in facing depression in all of its forms. And it is also dedicated to the healers who work with these patients. May you be filled with kindness and compassion and find ways to sustain yourselves over a lifetime of service.

You are all unsung heroes.

CONTENTS

The

CHEMISTRY

of

JOY

A Three-Step Program for Overcoming Depression
Through Western Science and Eastern Wisdom

1

THE MYSTERIOUS MIX OF
SCIENCE AND SPIRIT

Surely joy is the condition of life.
—HENRY DAVID THOREAU

Imagine for a moment a cardiologist seeing a new patient. The man smokes, is forty pounds overweight, and subsists on a diet of pizza, french fries, and Big Macs. He works at a stressful job that leaves him agitated at the end of every fourteen-hour day, and his most strenuous exercise is walking from his office to the parking lot. He has a family history of heart disease, and his blood pressure and cholesterol are through the roof.

"Okay," says the cardiologist after he reviews the results of the tests, conducted by the nurse and a junior associate. He himself has spent just ten minutes with this patient, and already he's late for his next appointment. "Here's something to help your cholesterol go down, and something for your pressure. You shouldn't have many side effects, though you might experience some memory problems, and, of course, a loss of sex drive. But I wouldn't worry about it. Good luck, and I'll see you in three months when your prescription runs out."

You don't even have to be a first-year medical student to see what's wrong with this picture. Wait a minute, you say. Why didn't the doctor tell his patient to stop smoking, eat better, get more exercise, and find some strategies for coping with stress? Why isn't he monitoring the patient more carefully? And why is the patient's only option medications that, while they may save his life, will make it even less pleasant?

At this point, we'd never think of treating heart disease in such a limited fashion. It may have taken a while, but both the medical community and the general public have finally adopted an integrated approach to this potentially fatal illness. Yet depression—once viewed entirely as a psychological or spiritual problem—is now treated almost exclusively with medication alone by the vast majority of the medical establishment. While it's hard to imagine the cardiologist who would treat a heart patient in the way I've described, some version of this scenario would be not at all unusual for a harried psychiatrist at an HMO, under pressure to find the quickest and most cost-effective treatment for depression, nor for the family doctors who prescribe antidepressants while ignoring their patients' diet, exercise, and lifestyle. Even responsible, caring physicians—psychiatrists as well as general practitioners—are unaware that depression requires a "brain-healthy" diet and lifestyle to mirror the "heart-healthy" regime that we've come to know so well. Even well-meaning psychiatrists tend to see depressed patients as brain chemistry gone awry rather than as a complex integration of mind, body, and spirit. And many patients who try to eat well, exercise frequently, and live a healthy life remain ignorant of the specific diet and lifestyle choices that might cure their insomnia, lift their moods, soothe their anxiety, and generally ease their depression.

Depression is a holistic illness that affects every aspect of who we are as human beings. It only makes sense to address it from every available angle, both with regard to our bodies and brain chemistry and vis-à-vis our psyches and spirits. So in this book, I offer you a revolutionary model for treating depression, one that integrates physical, mental, and spiritual approaches to help you discover "the chemistry of joy"—that mysterious mix of body, mind, and spirit that Thoreau called "the condition of life."

I believe that no matter how much pain each of us is given to endure—and for some of us, the burden is considerable—we can also always access the joy that is our birthright. But to find the joy we're all meant to experience, we need to understand ourselves fully, including our physical, emotional, and spiritual needs. A program for overcoming depression that omits any one of these aspects of our humanity is almost certain to fail.

A THREE-STEP PROGRAM TO CREATING JOY

My approach to overcoming depression and creating joy is based on two decades of work as a psychiatrist who has also studied Jungian psychology, Christian theology, Buddhist philosophy, Ayurvedic medicine, and the groundbreaking mindfulness approach to physical and mental health pioneered by Jon Kabat-Zinn and Saki Santorelli. In developing the program I'll share with you here, I've drawn on the latest developments in Western biochemistry to help me understand the elegant and complex interactions that take place constantly within our extraordinary brain. I've refined my understanding of diet, exercise, and lifestyle through the Ayurvedic Mind-Body medicine I learned from my study with Deepak Chopra. And I've deepened my approach to psychotherapy by incorporating a Buddhist Psychology of Mindfulness. Together, Western science and Eastern wisdom have enabled me to create this three-step program.

Step One: Understand Your Brain

Step One is your first line of defense against depression, the techniques to which you turn when you're in the throes of a depressive episode and need immediate help. It's based on the understanding that just as the heart patient needs a "heart-healthy lifestyle," so do depressed patients need a "brain-healthy" program that includes diet, exercise, and a healthy relationship to natural cycles—the ultradian, circadian, and seasonal rhythms that affect us more than we think.

Although by now even fast-food addicts have the guilty sense that french fries and pizza aren't exactly good for our health, very few of us realize that these poor food choices are also disastrous for our mood. Too many refined carbs and unhealthy fats play havoc with our brain chemistry as well as our weight, working against our efforts to overcome depression no matter how much medication we take.

Depending on our individual system, even apparently healthy diets can be bad for our brains. I recently met a man in his fifties who worked out regularly and had a lean, healthy physique. He ate mainly home-cooked, low-fat meals featuring high-quality proteins and fresh fruits and vegetables. But he wasn't getting the complex carbohydrates that he needed to overcome a lifelong serotonin deficiency, nor the healthy Omega-3 fats that his brain craved. As a result he suffered from anxiety, insomnia, and a tendency to depression. When he added more whole grains, legumes, and starchy vegetables into his diet, his mood, sleep, and well-being improved almost instantly. In Step One, you'll learn how to tell if you, too, are eating exactly the wrong foods to balance your brain chemistry, with concrete suggestions for how to switch to a "brain-healthy" diet.

Step One is also where I'll introduce three types that you'll continue to encounter throughout the book, although they may appear slightly different each time you meet them. One of the most exciting discoveries I've made in my practice is the way Western biochemistry, Ayurvedic Mind-Body medicine, and Buddhist psychology have all identified three distinct types, each of whom needs a different physical and emotional approach to overcoming depression. In Step One, we'll start with a Western scientific explanation, based on the balance of biochemicals in the brain. Our mood, energy level, and outlook are determined to a remarkable extent by the relationship between our levels of *serotonin*—a soothing chemical—and our supply of *dopamine* and *norepinephrine*, which stimulate us. When these chemicals go out of balance, we become depressed—but different types of imbalance result in different categories of depression, which seem in turn to be tied to different personality types:

- *Anxious Depression:* People with low levels of serotonin often feel fearful, inadequate, and nervous, always worried about the future and their own inability to measure up to life's demands. They tend to hold on too tightly and may become dependent in relationships.
- *Agitated Depression:* People with high levels of norepinephrine/dopamine, possibly combined with low levels of serotonin, frequently feel angry, resentful, bitter, and despairing. They're often judgmental, demanding, and highly critical in relationships, with a tendency to push away anyone who doesn't meet their high standards.
- *Sluggish Depression:* People with inadequate levels of norepinephrine and dopamine tend to slow down, sleep way too much, and have trouble concentrating or motivating themselves to work. When depressed, they often become confused and "absent," even—or perhaps especially—in their most intimate relationships.

Because Western scientists developed these categories in terms of depression, each description represents the most extreme, unhealthy versions of each type. But all of us have tendencies in one or more of these directions, whether we're talking about an occasional "blue day" or a diagnosis of clinical depression. Thus, all of us can benefit from the diet and lifestyle recommended for our "type," once we've identified which it is.

So in Step One, you'll find out what kind of diet your brain-chemistry type requires, as well as the exercise, daily schedule, and sleep patterns that can help keep your brain chemicals in balance. Even if you've never been diagnosed with depression or don't think of yourself as depressed, you can benefit from identifying your particular brain-chemistry needs and then following the recommendations in Step One.

Step Two: Make Use of Mind-Body Medicine

Step Two is your next line of defense against depression, a further effort to rebalance your system once you've begun making the diet and lifestyle changes in Step One. It's based on the principles of Ayurveda, an ancient system of Mind-Body medicine used for centuries in India and neighboring countries. Since this healing system has been around for several centuries, imagine my surprise when I realized that it basically offered more a spiritual and poetic version of the same three brain-chemistry types that Western medicine had identified—complete with diet and lifestyle suggestions that correspond with remarkable similarity to Western prescriptions.

When I began using these Mind-Body precepts to treat my patients, I discovered that they went beyond conventional science to help me fine-tune my recommendations for nutrition, exercise, and other brain-healthy activities that could help my patients rebalance their brain chemistry. As a result, I now routinely identify each of my patients' Ayurvedic type to help me better tailor my suggestions to their needs. When you take the quiz in Chapter 7, you can identify your own Ayurvedic type and go on to adopt the practices that are most beneficial for you.

Air Types are most prone to the Western disorder known as "anxious depression." People in this category are typically thin, wiry, and fine-boned—sensitive and quick. If you're an Air type, you're frequently on the move, like a breath of fresh air or a cooling wind. You're probably an excellent communicator, with an active mind that moves easily from one topic to the next. You may also have a tendency to be spacey and ungrounded, with difficulty digesting the knowledge you acquire—as well as the food you eat. Because Air types can exhaust their energy through overactivity, you need foods, spices, and activities that will help center and ground you. In fact, the diet that I'd recommend for a serotonin-deficient patient is remarkably similar to the nutritional advice for Air types in Ayurveda.

Fire Types, by contrast, are most vulnerable to the Western disorder known as "angry or agitated depression," marked by excess dopamine and norepinephrine, and probably with low serotonin levels as well. People in this category are usually well-muscled, warm, and energetic. If you're a Fire type, your friends would probably describe you as dynamic, sharp-witted, and "fiery," an active person who tends to engage in life with great enthusiasm and mental clarity. Yet your very sharpness can also make you irritable and angry, while your enthusiasm can morph into competitiveness. To soothe your fire, you need cooling, calming foods, activities, and spices. Once again, Ayurvedic prescriptions can fine-tune, extend, and enhance Western medical advice.

Earth Types are prone to "sluggish depression," caused by a shortage of the stimulating chemicals dopamine and norepinephrine. (People in this category may also suffer from a serotonin deficiency.) Earth types tend to be solid, large-boned, and fleshy. If you fit in this category, you're stable and earthy, the kind of person who is reliable and soothing to be around, the "earth mother" (or "earth father"!) on whom everyone tends to rely. However, your very stability can sometimes lead you to get stuck in a rut. So if you're an Earth type, you need stimulating foods, activities, and spices to stay motivated and active.

Combination Types: Some people are a combination of two Ayurvedic types, and so they need to figure out the diet, exercise plan, and activities that are most balancing for them. And some people partake of all three types. When these "triple combination" folks get depressed, they might suffer from anxiety, anger, *and* sluggishness, as their brain chemicals fluctuate and their mood varies.

Even if you fit clearly into a single type, these categories are not absolute. To some extent, we all share qualities from each type, just as many patients seem to blur the lines among Western categories of brain chemistry. But I've found it enormously useful to help my patients identify their basic types (or combinations) and to choose food, exercise, and activities accordingly, particularly when they're under stress, feeling out of balance, or struggling with a depressive episode.

Step Three: Understand the Psychology of Mindfulness

Once you've balanced your physical self with the suggestions in Steps One and Two, you can go on to the psychological and spiritual issues that can help you create a long-term strategy for overcoming depression and finding joy. Toward this end, I can recommend no better approach than *mindfulness*, the cornerstone of Buddhist psychology. The practice of mindfulness is based on the theory that the way to achieve joy in life—even in the midst of suffering—is to be *mindful*: aware, in the moment, and responding with intention.

Unfortunately, most of us fall short of that ideal much of the time. Instead of responding with intention, we react automatically, unconsciously, and often to issues in our past rather than to what is happening in the present moment. So prevalent is our tendency to respond with automatic reactions that Buddhist psychologists have identified three basic patterns of reactivity. Once again, I was astonished to discover that the Buddhist Emotional types correspond to both Western and Ayurvedic categories:

The Grasping or Fear Type: If you're prone to the Western diagnosis of "anxious depression/low serotonin," you're probably an Air type—and a Fear type. Your tendency is to react to stress with fear and anxiety, based on the worry that you're "not enough" and that the world doesn't contain enough to satisfy everyone. Your stress may also take the form of greed, envy, self-doubt, and feelings of inadequacy, all reflections of your core belief that you must constantly grasp after "more"—whether in the inner or outer realm. You have what the psychologists of mindfulness would call a "wanting mind," the feeling that if you could only *get* more or *be* more, you'd be safe and secure. To overcome the feeling that you're "not enough" and don't have enough, generosity is your special route to joy.

The Rejecting or Anger Type: This type corresponds to the Western biochemical pattern of excess norepinephrine and dopamine (and possibly also low serotonin), a condition usually diagnosed as agitated depression. In Mind-Body terms, you're a Fire type. In Psychology of Mindfulness terms, you have a judging mind, and when you're stressed, you often react with anger, frustration, aggression, or hostility. Your automatic, unconscious response to a setback is often seeking someone to blame—others, yourself, or both. Your path to joy involves developing the antidote to anger—compassion.

The Adrift or Denial Type: People who are prone to low dopa/norepi levels and "sluggish depression"—what Mind-Body medicine calls Earth types—are likely to react to stress with confusion. These are Denial types who feel frequently adrift. If you're a Denial type, you'll notice that difficult situations often inspire you to "turn off," "numb out," or freeze, seemingly without emotions or opinions. Awareness is your route to joy, waking up to life's many possibilities and to your own vital nature.

Although most of my patients have no interest in Buddhism per se, they've found it useful to think in terms of these types, and so have I. Whatever your religious or spiritual orientation—including those of you who have no particular interest in religion—I think you'll find these types useful as well. Knowing your Emotional type can help you identify patterns in your reactions to stress, while learning the Psychology of Mindfulness and the strategies it employs—meditation, conscious breathing, and other techniques—can empower you to choose wiser and more conscious responses.

As with the Mind-Body categories, you may find that you fit more than one Emotional type. You may also discover that in some situations, you tend to respond with fear, while others set off your anger, and still others provoke confusion. In that case, mindfulness offers you a whole repertoire of strategies to help you respond to whatever type of depression you're struggling with. But mindfulness offers far more than simply overcoming depression. It is also an important component in the chemistry of joy.

MY JOURNEY TOWARD MINDFULNESS

My own journey toward a more integrated approach to depression began almost as soon as I had entered medical school. To some extent, this effort to integrate physical, emotional, and spiritual treatments comes from a lifelong habit of liking to synthesize, to bring apparently separate concepts into a single, dynamic framework. But I also had a very practical reason for seeking a new approach. It seemed very clear to me, from the moment I began my studies, that our treatment of depression was sadly lacking. People were suffering, and the conventional approaches to their condition just couldn't help them—not enough. The kinds of medications that were offered, the kinds of therapy that were traditionally done, just weren't solving the problem. And the suffering went on.

Throughout my training, I'd sought for ways to integrate a psychological and spiritual approach into the predominantly biological worldview I encountered. I studied Jungian psychology, family systems, and a type of pastoral counseling called "spiritual direction," which I explored at a divinity school in Rochester, New York, the town where I was also doing my psychiatry training.

After I finished my residency, I returned to my native Midwest and took a job at a large HMO in Minneapolis, where I had the opportunity to treat literally hundreds of people. It was a fantastic learning experience—but I eventually came to see it as a rather industrialized approach to medicine. It ultimately wasn't satisfying for me, and I didn't think it was very good for my patients, either.

For a while, I joined another practice, but I kept encountering the same assembly-line mentality and reductionist philosophy. For a field that had begun with such a broad view of human nature, psychiatry seemed to have devolved into a mechanistic vision of brain chemicals and medications.

Then one day I happened to catch a Bill Moyers special called *Healing and the Mind*, featuring the pioneering work of Jon Kabat-Zinn. A researcher and scientist, Kabat-Zinn had realized that medical science was missing an important aspect of healing. He developed his "mindfulness-based stress reduction program," which eventually became an extraordinary eight-week course integrating Buddhist principles with medical science. Jon's focus was on chronic medical concerns, but I saw that his approach would be extremely helpful to psychiatric patients as well.

I was lucky enough to be one of the first doctors to train with Jon, who has gone on to teach his course to literally hundreds of physicians and health professionals. It's not an exaggeration to say that he and his colleague Saki Santorelli have transformed U.S. medicine, particularly as it approaches chronic diseases. Jon demonstrated that meditation could not only help reduce stress but could also affect the course of a disease, not to mention a patient's experience of his or her condition. I've spent over a decade now teaching mindfulness-based classes in all kinds of different settings. Gradually, I've developed the three-step method that I share in this book, an integration of Western biochemistry and Eastern wisdom that offers a radically new approach to overcoming depression.

Why is this integrated approach important? First, because the Western biochemical diagnosis, while crucial to understanding the nature of depression, goes only so far. Although we know something about the physical needs and personality types that corresponded to these biochemical categories, Western psychiatry's focus has become limited to an understanding of chemistry.

Second, each of the Eastern perspectives adds a different dimension to our understanding of the three types of depression. Ayurvedic Mind-Body typing is based on an elaborate set of dietary, exercise, and lifestyle prescriptions—recommendations that I soon found were of enormous help to my patients. Once I began thinking of my patients as Air, Fire, or Earth types, I could offer them suggestions that corresponded to but went far beyond Western-based recommendations for nutrition, exercise, and lifestyle. I could also bring a spiritual perspective to my suggestions, seeing Air types as needing to be grounded, Fire types as needing to be cooled and soothed, and Earth types as requiring stimulation and movement. I found this imagery helped me hear my patients' stories on a deeper level, while better directing my own attention to the question of what would help them restore balance in their lives. Even when I'd only considered Western biochemistry, I wanted to help my patients balance their brain chemistry. Now I was able to put that intention into a larger framework.

Likewise, having access to the Buddhist notions of Emotional types helped me to further articulate the issues with which my patients struggled. Buddhist psychology helped me form diagnoses even as it helped my patients approach their problems in a new way. While I continue to make use of the Western psychological tradition, I have come to rely equally on the notion of mindfulness and its focus on the observing self. If you can observe yourself—even in distress—without blame, without judgment, and then choose, calmly, a wise response to whatever situation you're in, you begin to see that depression, however painful, is not insurmountable. Helping my patients replace automatic, unconscious reactions with intentional, conscious responses has opened the door to many people who could not be helped by traditional psychotherapy—or who could be helped more when mindfulness was added to the mix.

Finally, integrating all three perspectives has enabled me to distinguish between a short- and a long-term approach to depression. Now when patients come to me in the throes of depression, I offer them immediate intervention in the form of physical changes—diet, exercise, supplements, and the like, as well as medications if they need them. I help them refine their lifestyle choices, using the well-articulated Ayurvedic Mind-Body system to extend their understanding of what their bodies need.

But the mental and spiritual aspects of Ayurveda are already pointing toward the future, in which Buddhist psychology and mindfulness practices can become a long-term strategy to prevent future episodes of depression by reorienting a person's entire worldview. To my mind, depression is a profound learning experience, offering us the opportunity to reconsider the choices we've made and strike out for new goals. But in order to be enlarged rather than diminished by the experience, we need a spiritual perspective. Buddhist psychology and the practice of mindfulness seemed to offer such an outlook.

THE ENEMIES OF JOY

The incidence of depression has been increasing at an alarming rate. According to the Cross-National Collaborative Group, the number of people struggling with depression has increased by about 10 percent every decade since 1910—and despite the pharmaceutical explosion of the past two decades, the increase shows no sign of slowing. If anything, the rate is going up faster than ever, making depression the leading cause of disability in the United States.

When I report this alarming statistic to the physicians, social workers, and other health professionals who attend my classes and workshops, I'll usually hear someone say, "Oh, it's not that depression itself is increasing, but only that people are reporting it more often."

But in fact, the statistics are not based on either patients' self-descriptions or doctors' diagnoses. Rather, researchers over the years have investigated the U.S. population from an epidemiological viewpoint—seeking evidence for the existence of depression out in the community rather than in statistics from clinics, doctors, or hospitals. The data come from a representative sampling of the population with whom researchers have done structured interviews designed to ferret out the symptoms of depression: low mood; impaired sleep and appetite; loss of energy, interest, motivation, and pleasure. In other words, no matter how individuals described their own psychological condition or whether they had ever been formally diagnosed, researchers have been able to infer that the incidence of depression was on the rise.

Not only is the rate of depression higher but it is occurring at an ever-earlier age. The problem is spreading worldwide, too, so that the World Health Organization (WHO) estimates that depression will be the single greatest cause of disability worldwide by the year 2020. WHO attributes the epidemic to the fact that more and more nations are "Westernizing." Clearly, something about our modern way of life is making us sick.

What, then, are the enemies of joy, the factors in our lives and our society that literally depress us? In my opinion, they are three:

1. ***Physical Imbalance and Toxicity.*** Even though I come from a psychological and spiritual perspective, as a physician, I can never ignore the role of the body. I know that we're all born with a certain genetic makeup that may cause more problems for some of us than others. Our inborn levels of resilience are simply different, and people with low levels of resilience can more easily fall into depression.

   But beyond what we're born with come the choices we make and the world we're surrounded by. The poor quality of food available to most of us—vegetables and fruits grown in mineral-depleted soil; animal products laced with hormones; processed foods laden with refined sugars and saturated in unhealthy fats; industrial, agricultural, and environmental toxins—threatens our mental as well as our physical health. Our brain is literally affected by the poisons that surround us, which promote inflammation, impede adrenal gland function, and burden our brain chemistry in a thousand different ways.

   As if that weren't enough, our speeded-up economic life subjects most of us to enormous levels of work-related stress, while the lack of social safety nets means that most of us are constantly worried about money. Lack of sleep, tension at home and at work, the insistence on a constant round of activity unrelieved by rest—all of these are major contributors to depression.

2. ***The Mind Runs Rampant.*** Depression is not only a disease of the body, however. It's also a disease of the mind. If our minds are allowed free rein, if they are allowed to run away with us, fretting endlessly over worries about the future, seething constantly with resentment against real or imagined grievances, or shutting down en-

tirely in response to stress, we will sooner or later pay the price in depression.

Moreover, most of us don't understand our mind's role in creating our emotions, our experience of life, our mood, and even our physical health. Our lack of awareness means that we can't find good strategies for dealing with our fearful, angry, or confused minds. Instead, we confuse our mind's perceptions with reality, and we allow our unwise mental strategies—worry, anxiety, blame, retaliation, denial, confusion—to determine the course of our lives. It's a depressing way to live—and we are, accordingly, depressed.

3. *The Illusion of Separation.* At the most profound level, we're only human in community. Think of a poor, isolated soul on a desert island, with no one to talk to for years at a time. Do you imagine that person—even if he or she never had to worry about food, shelter, or basic survival—would survive such an experience mentally, emotionally, and spiritually intact? It doesn't seem likely. We're meant to be part of one another's lives, and we need to share in each other's humanity. But in our modern culture, with its focus on individualism and separate achievement, we lose the sense of connectedness that keeps us sane—and depression is often the result.

It's not only connectedness to other humans that we need. We're part of the natural world, and losing that lifeline can also depress us more than we realize. We need, too, a link to the divine—to the universe itself—a sense of the higher purpose of which we are a part. Without the sense that the universe is a friendly place to which we belong as to a family, we have great difficulty not to become depressed.

I don't want to romanticize the past. Certainly the world has always been a violent and frightening place, and the extended families and tight-knit communities that once characterized most of humankind were often claustrophobic, repressive, and cruel. Perhaps there is no healthy alternative in the past—but that doesn't mean the present is healthy, either. Our isolated, alienated world is a breeding ground for depression—and the rapid rise of this painful disorder is the sad result.

Surrounded as we are by these enemies of joy, outside as well as within us, we need healing more than we ever have. In my observation, the kind of therapy usually offered in our modern system of HMOs and short-term treatments is simply not enough for many people. Given the crisis in our health-care system—a crisis that extends to both patients and the system itself—shouldn't we be looking for creative solutions to these thorny problems? Integrating Western science with Eastern wisdom is my own attempt to find a new paradigm within which we might seek healing.

THE CHEMISTRY OF JOY

When I first explained my three-step program to my patient Melanie, she balked at considering her depression in terms of brain chemistry. "I hate thinking of myself as just a collection of chemicals," she told me bluntly. "I'd like to feel as though I had more control over my life and emotions than that. 'Put in one chemical, and I'll react one way; put in another chemical and I'll react another way'—it makes me feel as though I'm just some puppet, some victim of my own brain."

My patient Martin had the opposite reaction. A man with a great respect for science, Martin found profound relief in understanding the role that physical factors played in his depression. But he didn't understand why I suggested that he meditate, practice conscious breathing, and engage in "heart-opening" exercises.

"Just prescribe me the meds I need, tell me what to eat, and I'll be on my way," Martin told me. "I'm not interested in all that spiritual mumbo jumbo."

I tried to explain to both Melanie and Martin that my approach was based in an integration of body, mind, and spirit. Indeed, my best understanding *as a scientist* is that how we feel, what we eat, the choices we make, and the levels of biochemicals in our brains are all profoundly interactive. True, low levels of the chemical serotonin are correlated with certain types of depression, as we'll see in Chapter 2. But what causes the low levels of serotonin? Diet, genetic background, exercise habits, life events, early childhood experiences, and our daily habits of thought all play a role in the level of this vital chemical in our brains. Moreover, each of these factors affects every other factor. The right diet can give us more energy to exercise; a new meditation may motivate us to change our diet; a productive therapy session can, at least temporarily, flood our brains with helpful chemicals indicating that, at least for a while, we've found a measure of calm and well-being.

Likewise, Martin's resistance to "mumbo jumbo," while understandable, leaves out the profoundly transformative role that our thoughts, feelings, and beliefs can have on our brain chemistry. To take a trivial example, consider the experience of a long, boring, indefinite wait, perhaps in a stuffy airport or out under the blazing summer sun. Standing in line under such circumstances can be excruciating if our thoughts have nothing better to do than bubble with annoyance—and our serotonin levels would drop accordingly, in response to the heat and stress.

Now imagine the same long wait with a long-lost friend or a fascinating mystery novel to help you pass the time. Suddenly your awareness of the physical discomfort vanishes because your mind has another focus. And the pleasure you take in talking or reading will likewise be reflected in your brain chemistry.

So when we think of all the different factors that go into creating or overcoming our depression, we should think less of a row of dominoes, set off by a single push, and more of a complicated pinball machine in which several balls are released in response to the first pull of the trigger. Picture the way a pinball machine seems to take on a life of its own, the way each little movement of the ball triggers a half-dozen other bells, lights, and new balls. You don't have complete control over what happens—if you shake or hit the machine, it will simply turn off. But you do have some control over keeping the balls in play, and you can learn—at least to some extent—to "dance" with all the simultaneous actions instead of trying to slow down and analyze each event.

Our brains—and our lives—are more complicated than any pinball machine, and we're only beginning to understand all the different factors that create our energy, our well-being, and our mood. In this book, you'll have the opportunity to learn more about some of what I've come to consider the key factors—brain chemistry, diet, exercise, mental outlook, and openness of spirit. Working with any one of these factors can make a huge difference in overcoming your depression. Working with all of them at once can create a kind of quantum improvement that may, over time, astonish you. This potential for both slow transformation and quantum leaps is to me the true value of the chemistry of joy.

STEP ONE

Understand Your Brain

2

BASIC BRAIN CHEMISTRY

When I first met my patient Dave, I was tempted to say he'd been living a blessed life. Dave had grown up in a large, loving family of high achievers, the child of highly successful parents. He and his siblings—with the exception of one mildly depressed brother—went on to achieve similar success, and even that brother enjoyed a healthy marriage, loving children, and financial success. Unlike many families I knew, Dave's had remained close and supportive even as the children grew into adulthood, and the extended family of in-laws, nieces, and nephews remained equally warm and connected.

Dave married a schoolteacher with whom he'd raised two lovely children, both in high school, by the time I met him. Although he worked long hours in his financial planning and brokerage business, he'd always prided himself on his stamina, and he generally enjoyed both the work itself and the challenges of succeeding in such a competitive field. He and his wife had an active social life with many close friends, and he was active in his community as well.

Yet as Dave approached fifty, the problems began to pile up. First, his mother died; then Dave's sister suddenly got a divorce from his favorite brother-in-law. Dave took a serious hit in the economic downturn and found his work growing more stressful and competitive. Most painful, though, was being called at work one day about his son. The teenage boy had been caught with marijuana, and the resulting investigation led to his suspension from school.

As Dave told me his story, I realized that he was concerned about his mood for the first time in his life. He felt disheartened, bereft of the optimism he'd always counted on before. His family had started to complain about how irritable he was, how short-tempered. Also for the first time, he was having trouble sleeping. Even when he managed to get eight hours, he'd wake up feeling low-energy and listless, dragging himself through a long day at work. Then, at night, he'd feel restless and agitated. Finally, he went to his family doctor, hoping to get something to help him sleep. Luckily, his physician referred him to me.

I explained to Dave that he was suffering from mild depression, probably related to low levels of serotonin, a key biochemical found in the brain and the gut. I suggested that rather than medicate one of his symptoms—sleeplessness—we start by trying to shift this chemical balance.

Dave looked at me in confusion. "But I've never been depressed in my life," he told me. "If I had a problem with brain chemistry, wouldn't it have shown up by now?"

REFILLING THE FOUNTAIN: RESILIENCE, BIOCHEMISTRY, AND DEPRESSION

Dave's story illustrates one of the most important concepts in our understanding of depression: *resilience*. In this key notion lies an explanation for why some of us are depressed constantly; others become depressed in response to seemingly minor incidents; and still others seem able to withstand one difficult circumstance after another without depression.

Imagine that inside each of us, there is a container like one of those watercoolers you find in every office—a large jug that opens at the press of a valve. Our container is full of a magic liquid—a fountain of resilience—that keeps us afloat when times get tough. At the first sign of any trouble, challenge, or excitement, the container releases some of that blessed elixir to soothe, comfort, or protect our stressed-out brain.

Every time we encounter a stressful situation—from the mild challenge of being late for an appointment to the major stressor of a parent's or spouse's illness—the levels in our tank drop. Eventually, after the challenge has passed, our fountain will replenish itself and the tank will refill. When it's full, we're relaxed and content. When it's half-full, we're mildly depressed, agitated, or stressed out. And when our tank is nearly empty, the fountain run dry, we're severely depressed.

The important thing to remember here is that everyone's tank emp-
ties and refills—but at a different rate. All of us will experience depression and/or anxiety when our chemical levels fall too low. But the
amount of stress it takes to lower those levels—and to keep them
down—is different in every one of us.

To continue with our metaphor, it's as though we're genetically en-
dowed with containers of different sizes. People like Dave may be able
to withstand several major stressors before the chemicals in their tank
sink to a dangerous level. People born with lower resilience might find
that a relatively minor setback—or simply the stresses of getting
through the day—can precipitate a serious depression.

But even Dave has his limits. And in the wake of his mother's
death, his sister's divorce, his son's disgrace, and his increasingly difficult
workload, he begins to face a noticeably empty tank for the first time in
his life. Dealing with all these stresses has used up too many of the crucial chemicals in Dave's brain, lowering them to a dangerous level, and
he's had neither the time nor the resources to replenish them. That's
why he's experiencing sleeplessness, irritability, agitation, and listlessness for the first time in his life. Until he encountered this unusual degree of stress, his "full tank"—his naturally high resilience—had kept
these symptoms at bay.

Dave's generally high resilience contrasts strongly with the naturally
low resilience of my patient Jennifer. I first met Jennifer in October, two
months into her freshman year of college. This talented young woman
was a good student and a gifted musician, but she'd had a hard time in
high school, struggling to fit in and keep her spirits up. Jennifer's alcoholic father had left when she was in middle school. Jennifer continued
to live with her mother, whom she considered her best friend. But leaving for college was something of a relief, partly because her mom was so
negative and depressed all the time.

Jennifer had entered her top-rated competitive college full of excitement, ready for a fresh start. She had particularly high hopes for her
social life, thinking that she'd find other bright, artistic kids to hang out
with and date. But by October, her initial enthusiasm had waned. She
was used to being at the top of her class in high school, and now she felt
fairly average academically. Nor had she generated any obvious interest
from boys. Slowly, her old self-doubts came creeping back.

One night, Jennifer's roommate and two of their friends went out without asking her to join them. She immediately felt abandoned and spent the whole evening brooding about what had happened. By the time her roommate returned at 2 a.m., Jennifer was crying helplessly in her bed.

As we saw, Dave didn't encounter even mild depression until he'd undergone three family crises and a major downturn at work. Jennifer, by contrast, was in the throes of fairly serious depression after relatively minor trouble at school and one upsetting incident with a friend. Clearly the levels in her "tank" had already fallen significantly before she ever experienced her first symptom. Indeed, her family history—a depressed mother and a father who might have "self-medicated" his depression by drinking—suggested that Jennifer may have been born with a genetic predisposition to depression: a small and easily emptied tank.

We're guaranteed to encounter some pain in this life. The good news is that there's quite a bit we can do to keep our fountains full, overflowing with the soothing chemicals that can help us cope with whatever challenges life throws us. No matter what size container we're born with—whether we're naturally resilient, like Dave, or less so, like Jennifer—all of us can keep our brain chemicals balanced through diet, exercise, lifestyle, and meditation.

OUR INTRICATE BRAINS

Of course, the idea of the tank is only a metaphor. But our brains really do require baseline levels of certain biochemicals to function properly. And when these levels get too low, or when our brains contain the wrong proportions of these chemicals, we often experience depression, anxiety, and even the urge to suicide.

Let's take a closer look. The brain is a vastly complicated web of nerve cells, or neurons, all poised to transmit mental messages as the brain communicates with itself. Moreover, chemical messengers—hormones and neuropeptides—can send signals from the brain to the rest of the body, instructing us via the bloodstream to feel strong and energized, calm and relaxed, or sluggish and bloated.

At the same time, chemicals produced in the gut, the heart, and our other organs also travel through the bloodstream, sending messages to the brain. Thus, when we feel agitated, we may have trouble digesting our food. On the other hand, when we eat a rich, hard-to-digest dinner, we might find it difficult to think clearly. Our bodies and brains affect each other, all the time.

Our brains are so elegant and complex that our understanding of them is still in its infancy. But we do know that thoughts, feelings, and sensations all work together; that the brain, gut, and other organs are continually interacting; and that your understanding of the world and of your own situation has an enormous impact on your mood, energy, and physical condition. Thus, understanding brain chemistry is one way of grasping how diet, exercise, genetics, and mental outlook all work together to create or overcome depression.

MOOD MESSENGERS: NEURONS AND NEUROTRANSMITTERS

How does the brain communicate with itself? The answer lies in the billions of neurons within our brains. Each of these neurons is capable of producing a little electromagnetic charge that travels from the heart of the neuron out to its edge until it reaches the fatty membrane that surrounds the cell. In order for your nerve cells to function properly, these membranes must be healthy, flexible, and adaptable, nourished with the right kinds of fats and proteins. (In Chapter 4, we'll find out more about what exactly you've got to eat in order to sustain these vital portions of your brain.) If your cell membrane is healthy, the electrical charge passes along it easily—but then it encounters a new obstacle.

Although our billions of neurons all work together, each is also a discrete entity, separated from its neighbors by a microscopic space called a synapse. The electricity that can travel freely within each cell stops short when it reaches the empty space between the cells. For the brain to transmit messages from one neuron to another, it needs chemical messengers, known as *neurotransmitters*, to jump the gap.

So the electrical impulse of the first neuron stimulates the cell to release a bit of neurotransmitter, which floats across the synapse to the next neuron. That second neuron receives the chemical message—which stimulates a new electrical charge. This second electrical impulse travels across the second cell, stimulating a second burst of neurotransmitter, which then crosses the third synapse, setting off the same process in the next cell. This whole chain of communication—electricity traveling across nerve cells; chemical messengers floating across synapses—happens literally as fast as thought itself, and it's not really such a linear journey. Whenever you think, feel, or experience a physical sensation, neurons are firing simultaneously all over your brain, generating a host of new thoughts, feelings, memories, and physical responses. (Remember our image of the pinball machine from Chapter 1.) You need healthy neurons and a good supply of neurotransmitters to keep this process working smoothly.

BRAIN CHEMICALS AND TYPES OF DEPRESSION

So what happens when one or more neurotransmitters is lacking? Then your brain will have difficulty sending and receiving messages. Likewise, if your neurotransmitters are out of balance—too much of some, not enough of others—your brain won't be able to process thoughts, information, and sensations the way it should. Symptoms of depression and anxiety—sleeplessness, hopelessness, worry, misery, and confusion—may be the result.

Thus, low levels of such neurotransmitters as serotonin, dopamine, and norepinephrine are the biochemical basis of anxiety and depression, whether the levels of these chemicals are naturally low, as for Jennifer, or have fallen in response to a series of crises, as for Dave. That's why a psychiatrist's first task is often to determine which chemicals are out of balance.

Unfortunately, no routine tests exist that can measure levels of brain chemicals—at least, not yet. But we can infer these levels by the types of depression and the clusters of symptoms that people manifest. Depending on which chemicals are imbalanced, you may tend toward *anxious depression*, *agitated depression*, or *sluggish depression*, each of which is a relatively distinct syndrome with its own behaviors and personality characteristics.

SEROTONIN AND ANXIOUS DEPRESSION

Serotonin is sometimes nicknamed the "well-being" chemical. Appropriate levels of this vital neurotransmitter help create feelings of peace, security, confidence, happiness, and joy. Imbalances are implicated not only in depression, but also in insomnia, migraine, premenstrual syndrome, and addiction, which may be why these conditions are often found in the same families, or, often, in the same people.

Serotonin sometimes operates like our brain's "responsible adult," helping us to "just say no" to impulsive behaviors such as aggression, binge eating, indiscriminate sexual activity, excessive gambling, and substance abuse. Studies have shown that people with low levels of serotonin may be more vulnerable to addictions and compulsive behavior, including alcoholism, drug addiction, compulsive shopping, and compulsive gambling. Likewise, a diet rich in serotonin-producing foods has been shown to help compulsive eaters resist the temptation to binge.

Besides being a "responsible adult," I also think of serotonin as our own personal "good parent," since whenever we feel worry, stress, or physical pain, our bodies release comforting levels of serotonin to help us cope. Thus, people with low levels of serotonin may have difficulty soothing or calming themselves, so that once a troubling thought or difficult event occurs, they may not be able to interrupt the anxiety or depression that results. Jennifer, for example, may have been unable to find relief from the misery of being left behind by her friends in part because of low serotonin levels. Once the blow occurred, she literally didn't have the resources to recover from it.

As with virtually every other aspect of our brains and bodies, serotonin levels are partly genetic, partly the result of early childhood experiences, and partly the outcome of our current choices in diet, exercise, and lifestyle. Children who grow up in warm, nurturing families, like Dave, may develop larger reserves of serotonin than people like Jennifer, with her divorced parents, depressed mother, and alcoholic father. Whenever Dave's mother or father soothed, comforted, or protected him, Dave experienced a rush of serotonin in response to the happy event. Thus he literally trained his brain to produce serotonin easily and often, which conditioned him to maintain high baseline serotonin levels. These high levels stood him in good stead throughout most of his life, enabling him to bounce back from stressful experiences and to maintain a generally high level of optimism and well-being.

Jennifer, on the other hand, grew up in a much more stressful environment. When her parents fought, or stopped speaking, or when her mother withdrew into depression, Jennifer had to draw on her own stores of serotonin to cope with the difficulties. Continually using up her serotonin in response to stress, she grew used to a much lower baseline level of the chemical, so that even small stresses could exhaust her already depleted stores.

The good news for Dave, Jennifer, and the rest of us is that there's a lot we can do to change our serotonin levels, both as a short-term response and as a long-term baseline. While Jennifer may always have to work harder than Dave to stay balanced, calm, and happy, she can do quite a bit to raise her baseline levels once she understands the problem. And high-resilience people like Dave can learn to recognize situations in which their serotonin levels are likely to be depleted, and take steps to keep them high.

Low levels of serotonin are probably implicated in all types of depression, at least to some extent. But when the major imbalance involves insufficient serotonin, you're likely to end up with some version of anxious depression, characterized by fear, anxiety, low self-esteem, and a host of related symptoms.

Symptoms of Serotonin Deficiency or "Anxious Depression"

- sad, irritable, or very changeable mood
- poor tolerance of stress; easily frazzled
- sensitive to criticism or rejection; low self-esteem
- dependent relationships
- impulsivity
- low blood sugar, binge eating, and carbohydrate craving
- anxiety, fearfulness, insomnia
- sensitivity to changes in biorhythm:
  - low winter light (seasonal affective disorder, or SAD)
  - monthly cycles (premenstrual syndrome, or PMS)
  - erratic sleep: jet lag or shift work
- alcohol abuse or family history of alcoholism
- excessive sweating, heat intolerance
- chronic pain
- impulsive or indiscriminate choice of multiple sexual partners
- suicidal thoughts or gestures

NOREPINEPHRINE, DOPAMINE, AND AGITATED DEPRESSION

If serotonin soothes us, norepinephrine and dopamine wake us up. These two brain chemicals are known as the "energizers." They help create alertness, energy, and aggression, and, accordingly, their lack creates sluggishness, listlessness, and passivity. As you might expect, stimulants like caffeine, cocaine, and "speed" temporarily induce the release of these vital chemicals, whereas alcohol, tranquilizers, and other depressants cue our bodies to make less of them.

When we're speaking casually, we often say something like, "That news gave me a huge shot of adrenaline," or "When I realized I only had ten minutes left to finish the report, I got a big adrenaline rush." In fact, adrenaline is a hormone that operates on the muscles, lungs, and bloodstream; dopamine and norepinephrine do the equivalent jobs in our brain. All three of these chemicals are present whenever we feel keyed up, excited, and ready for a fight. They are literally the "fight-or-flight" hormones that nature gave us to meet the most basic challenges to our survival. People with temporarily or naturally high levels of these chemicals feel strong, vital, and blessed with a great sense of personal power. Their thoughts move more quickly, and they're ready to respond in an instant to any new development.

Clearly, we need these energizing chemicals to stay alert, focused, and moving toward our goals. But too much of a good thing can be a problem—and excessive norepi and dopa levels, particularly combined with low serotonin, can produce a condition known as *agitated depression*. If you're suffering from this disorder, you're often angry, irritable, restless, and resentful. Nothing feels right, everyone disappoints you, and you can't seem to settle into a happy routine, a calm relationship, or an enjoyable work life. If your serotonin levels are low, or fluctuating, you may alternate between periods of intense restlessness and resentment, and times of hopelessness and misery.

Symptoms of Excess Dopamine/Norepinephrine, or "Agitated Depression"

- restlessness
- excessive energy, possibly alternating with periods of exhaustion or sluggishness
- anger and irritability
- flashes of unexpected temper and/or continual feelings of resentment
- sleep difficulties
- indigestion and acid stomach
- high blood pressure, possible increased risk of heart disease

---

NOREPINEPHRINE, DOPAMINE, AND SLUGGISH DEPRESSION

Have you ever gotten buzzed on too much coffee—and then crashed? Operating too long on a dopa/norepi "high" eventually exhausts our store of these energizing substances, and suddenly we, too, are exhausted. People with insufficient stores of dopa/norepi have often used up their stores of these vital chemicals from undergoing prolonged levels of stress or chronically stressful situations. For a while, our bodies may be up to the challenge, and some of us may even find it stimulating. Rescue workers and emergency-room nurses, for example, talk about the rush they get from coping with the hugely demanding situations into which their jobs thrust them every day.

Eventually, though, too much unrelieved stress over too long a time leaves us without any reserves to draw on. For those of us used to operating at a high level, the crash can seem to come suddenly and without warning, adding psychological distress and bewilderment to the physical and hormonal exhaustion.

Interestingly, strenuous physical exercise has an excellent "double effect" on our dopa/norepi levels. When you start to jog, bicycle, or lift weights, you may notice that your sluggish mood dissipates and you feel energized, powerful, and alert. That's because the mere act of using your muscles cues your brain to release more dopa/norepi into your system, and your hormone levels rise. Then the prolonged exercise uses up these fight-or-flight chemicals, so that after your workout, you feel relaxed. (We'll talk more about using exercise to prevent and overcome depression in Chapter 6.)

Either positive or negative situations can produce a rush of these energizing hormones. They can be released by the excitement of falling in love, landing a great new job, riding a roller coaster, or attending a rock concert. They can also be induced by the stress of coping with a looming work deadline, standing up to an abusive boss, or caring for a suddenly ill spouse. Any situation that is challenging, threatening, or exciting will set off a flood of dopa/norepi. Likewise, any type of exertion—physical, emotional, mental, or some combination thereof—will eventually deplete our dopa/norepi stores. Before we are ready to respond to the next challenge—or even to enjoy the next exciting treat—we'll have to replenish our chemical supplies.

Symptoms of Dopamine/Norepinephrine Depletion, or "Sluggish Depression"

- depressed mood
- low energy
- muscle problems (e.g., Parkinson's disease)
- increased sleep
- weight gain
- withdrawal, passivity
- decreased sex drive, impotence
- slowed thoughts, poor memory
- suicidal feelings

THE ROOTS OF DEPRESSION

When I talked with Jennifer about the role of brain chemistry in her depression, she was at first a bit confused. Even though she knew several people on antidepressants, she'd tended to think of medication as a mood-altering drug, something that would make her feel relaxed or happy almost against her will. Since she also knew several people in therapy, she herself tended more toward a psychological understanding of her condition. "I need to get in touch with my feelings, right? And then learn that I'm really not such a bad person after all?" she told me with more than a touch of teenage sarcasm.

I began by explaining my personal philosophy to Jennifer. Genetic "givens," early childhood experiences, and current diet and lifestyle choices all play a role in depression, I told her. So do our mental outlook, our understanding of ourselves and the world, and our ability to cope with our feelings. Certainly "talk therapy," as it's come to be called, can be a powerful aid in overcoming depression, and if she wanted to sign up for counseling sessions with me, I was happy to accept her as a patient. But I would be irresponsible not to help her understand the biochemical basis for her condition, especially since I had reason to think that her depression in particular had genetic roots.

"I know my mom is unhappy a lot of the time, but no one ever said she was 'depressed,' " Jennifer protested. "And my dad—forget it. He's a loud, cheerful guy, and when he's drinking, he's even more like that."

I told Jennifer that from her descriptions, both of her parents probably were depressed, even though neither had ever been formally diagnosed. Genetics probably accounts for 40 to 50 percent of mood disorders, including depression, but because mental illness has been stigmatized for so long, many people who today would be considered depressed have never been diagnosed.

If you think you might be suffering from depression, especially long-term, severe, or chronic depression, take another look at your family tree. My rural Minnesota patients come from a culture that prides itself on stoicism, so that even family members who have actively sought treatment for depression may not have shared this information with their children or siblings. But when I ask my patients about family patterns, I often hear such statements as "My mother spent a lot of time in her room crying," "My father was always irritable and moody," or "Grandma was one of the most negative people I've ever known—she always looked on the dark side."

Likewise, whenever I hear about a family history of alcohol abuse, I now consider it the same as a history of depression. And of course, if anyone in your family ever committed or attempted suicide, that's generally an indication of depression as well, even if no one ever spoke of it that way.

So, I told Jennifer, she'd come into this world with what was likely a genetic predisposition to depression. This didn't mean she was *destined* to become depressed—only that she had to be careful always to "keep her tank full."

However, given Jennifer's apparently low resilience and family history, she probably couldn't rely on talk therapy alone. Almost certainly she would need some kind of biological intervention, though not necessarily medication. Diet, nutritional supplements, exercise, and conscious breathing might be enough to boost her production of serotonin and other brain chemicals.

Jennifer listened thoughtfully to my explanation of high and low resilience, focusing with particular intensity on my description of how brain chemical baselines are often set in childhood. Then she asked what I considered a wonderful question: "Okay, so I've probably got a low baseline—is there anything I can do to make it higher?"

Yes, I told her, that was an excellent way to approach her situation. Not only could she cope on a short-term basis with the factors that had set off her current depression, she could look at a long-term plan involving diet, exercise, and meditation, possibly supplemented by talk therapy. A combination of physical, mental, and emotional approaches could indeed alter Jennifer's brain chemistry over time—perhaps not giving her the same degree of resilience that Dave was born with, but certainly boosting the resilience that *she* was born with. Raising her baseline level of brain chemicals might take a long time, and she might be in for a kind of back-and-forth process in which victories alternated with temporary setbacks. But if she was patient with herself and committed to this approach, she might be surprised at how much stronger and more resilient she could become. After all, a seed planted several inches below the ground might need longer to sprout than a seed dropped just below the earth's surface. But with time, patience, and care, both plants can break through to the sunlight.

3

THE PROMISE AND PERILS
OF MEDICATION

"I don't want to go on medication!" my patient Sarah said to me, almost in tears. "I've seen what it's done to my mother. She went on antidepressants ten years ago, and it's always the same—they work great for a few months, then they don't, and then she's worse. Then the doctor puts her on some new medication, and the whole thing starts all over again."

Sarah was unusual among my patients, many of whom come to me eager for the antidepressants about which they've heard so much. Both physicians and psychiatrists have come to view such medications as Paxil, Zoloft, and Wellbutrin as true "wonder drugs," medicines that have succeeded where traditional talk therapy and other approaches have failed. Even Prozac, despite the rash of bad publicity that it got for a while, continues to enjoy a reputation as a cure-all for anxiety and depression.

But Sarah's mother's predicament—a long-term reliance on medications that often work best only in the short term—is all too common, even if these more mundane problems of antidepressants don't get the public attention of the notorious suicides and psychotic episodes that were associated with Prozac in the early 1990s. Although I do prescribe antidepressants to my patients who need them, I also feel concerned about what I see as the overreliance on medication among psychiatrists, primary-care doctors, and other health professionals. For some people, antidepressants may indeed be a kind of wonder drug, balancing their brain chemistry and enabling them to take a new approach to their lives. But in many cases, these patients might benefit from alternatives to medication that will work just as well or better, with longer-term benefits and fewer side effects. And people who do need medications, whether temporarily or for a longer time, also need to support their brain chemistry in other ways, such as with nutrition, supplements, exercise, and breathing—approaches that all too many doctors and psychiatrists fail to recommend.

So in this chapter, I'll walk you through the promise and the perils of medication. I'll show you how these medications work and why they need to be supported with the right nutrition, exercise, and lifestyle. I'll tell you about alternatives to medication and help you evaluate whether they might be right for you. And if you're currently taking or about to take medications, I'll show you how you can work with your doctor or psychiatrist toward either getting off your antidepressants or making the best possible use of them over the long term.

> **Warning:** Antidepressants are very powerful medications that affect your brain chemistry, mood, and emotion in profound and long-lasting ways. You must NEVER attempt to stop taking them without the support of a doctor or psychiatrist, and you must NEVER stop taking them suddenly or try to reduce your dosage on your own. Agitation, disorientation, severe depression, and suicidal feelings are only some of the symptoms that might result from an improper cessation of antidepressants. This chapter is intended only to help you work with a qualified physician to make informed decisions about medication. Please do not interpret anything in this chapter as suggesting that you should reduce your dosage or alter your use of medication in any way without a doctor's supervision.

THE PRESCRIPTION REVOLUTION

When I was first learning to practice psychiatry, the pharmacological repertory was fairly limited. The standard treatment for depression was to prescribe one of two classes of drugs, MAO inhibitors and tricyclic antidepressants. Although both were somewhat effective in relieving the symptoms of depression, each brought with it such severe and uncomfortable side effects that for many patients, the cure was often worse than the disease.

Then came the new class of antidepressants, and it seemed like a miracle. These new medications were significantly more specific in rebalancing only those aspects of brain chemistry whose imbalance was causing depression.

The new effectiveness of antidepressants meant that many people who had been suffering from low-grade depression—perhaps without even realizing it—were suddenly taking these medications and feeling better. Today's antidepressants have even fewer side effects than that first generation of "miracle drugs," and the newest medicines are safer still. People take them and feel better almost immediately, which is a powerful reinforcer to keep taking them. And of course, the alternative—ongoing depression—is both upsetting to the patient and disturbing to the therapist, who is only too aware that suicide is a possible outcome of depression. "Better safe than sorry" becomes the slogan, and medications are almost generally viewed by my profession as entailing few shortcomings while delivering a significant number of benefits.

Today, tens of millions of Americans are now on antidepressants, and the number goes up each year. The cost of these prescriptions—at least five hundred dollars per person per year—is straining the health-insurance industry and is one of the reasons for health care's annual double-digit inflation.

This remarkable increase in the use of antidepressants is largely the result of a major educational effort of the past ten years, in which both medical schools and pharmaceutical companies have endeavored to train physicians to better recognize depression and to treat the condition with medication. When this effort began, I thought of it as a noble undertaking, even though much of it was funded by an industry that stood to make a handsome profit from these newly enlightened physicians. After all, when most people experience the first symptoms of depression, they start by going to their doctor, seeking advice on why they're so tired all the time or perhaps asking for medication to help them sleep. In fact, the vast majority of antidepressants are now prescribed by primary-care providers such as family physicians and nurse practitioners, and getting a prescription for an antidepressant is even easier than obtaining a flu shot. People who report symptoms of sleeplessness, agitation, or loss of energy to their family doctors—symptoms like the ones Dave presented to me—are likely to find their doctor suggesting a course of Paxil or Zoloft.

In some cases, this may be the right solution. Some people need the extra support that medication can provide to make it through a rough time or to combat what may be a lifelong tendency to depression. As we saw in Chapter 2, depression corresponds to an imbalance in brain chemistry, whether that imbalance results from a long-term pattern, childhood experience, genetic inheritance, or a specific situation. Whatever the cause, sometimes you just need medication to help restore your chemical balance.

But even when we focus entirely on the brain's chemistry, ignoring the many mental, emotional, and spiritual aspects of depression, medications often aren't the best way of rebalancing our hormones and biochemicals. Sometimes a change in diet and exercise habits can be equally effective, with no risk of side effects and with lifelong benefits to physical and mental health. Likewise, the approaches I describe in Step Three of this book have helped many of my patients overcome depression, both in response to specific causes or as part of a lifetime of unhappiness.

But even when medications are called for, doctors are often remiss in not prescribing the diet and lifestyle that would enable the meds to do their best work. As we saw in Chapter 1, practitioners who in other circumstances would not think of prescribing drugs without some lifestyle supports seem to consider antidepressants to be an end in themselves. Although no responsible physician would prescribe Lipitor without instructing the patient to cut back on fried foods, most doctors think nothing of prescribing Zoloft without an admonition to eat more complex carbs, cut out the sugar and caffeine, and get some vigorous exercise.

SARAH'S SEROTONIN SHORTAGE

Sarah was a young woman who had grown up in a small town and was now in college. She'd always struggled with a lack of confidence, she told me, and often felt insecure and anxious. Although Sarah was easily overwhelmed by stress, she actually had more difficulty with the times when she was less busy, when her chronic, low-grade sadness seemed to become more intense. Frequently, Sarah told me, she'd experience a day or two of inordinate sadness before her mood seemed to lift.

Sarah's mother had also suffered from depression, so Sarah was well aware that her symptoms were the classic ones for the condition. In the two weeks before she came to see me, Sarah's depression seemed to get worse, as she found herself crying frequently for no apparent reason. Sarah was also suffering from mild insomnia, feeling physically restless, and having trouble concentrating. Although she'd once loved her courses in history and art, she found herself losing interest in these favorite subjects, and it was becoming increasingly harder to motivate herself to study or even to attend class.

Sarah was used to struggling with periodic feelings of anxiety, hopelessness, and worthlessness. But now these emotions had intensified as well. Luckily, she was not suicidal. But she was experiencing virtually every other symptom of serotonin imbalance.

From having observed her mother's encounters with doctors over the years, Sarah was well aware that most mental-health professionals would diagnose her with major depression and prescribe an antidepressant. I was able to confirm that Sarah's family history of depression, her long-standing struggles with energy and mood, and her classic symptoms indicated a genetic tendency to low resilience. I agreed, too, that most doctors would very likely prescribe an antidepressant, most likely one of the class known as selective serotonin reuptake inhibitors, or SSRIs—Prozac, Zoloft, or Paxil. Indeed, someone with Sarah's symptoms would probably respond very well to that type of medication and feel much better almost immediately. So why not just prescribe it and give her some relief?

"If you were feeling suicidal," I told Sarah frankly, "or if you'd been feeling this low for a longer period—say, several weeks—I would almost certainly suggest that you consider medications. But in this case, you're absolutely right—there are lots of reasons not to rush to that step."

While the new medications are a vast improvement over the older class of antidepressants, I told her, even they can cause some side effects. In the early stages of treatment, patients often experience nausea, headaches, muscle tension, jitteriness, and insomnia, although these symptoms tend to improve over time, and they can be lessened if the dose is kept low and the medications are taken with food. Likewise, some patients—including, apparently, Sarah's mother—complain of feeling "flat," apathetic, or listless, though I consider those responses, too, a sign that the dosage is too high and needs to be adjusted.

Even if a medication is administered in the proper dosage, however, many patients experience long-term side effects such as weight gain, fatigue, and loss of libido—problems made worse by the fact that doctors often don't recognize these symptoms as side effects. Sometimes they're even considered evidence of lingering depression, with the result that the doctor increases the dosage of antidepressant and makes the problem worse.

Sarah's mother had also experienced the opposite problem—becoming more angry or agitated while on medications. Because of her mother's experience, Sarah was particularly anxious about recent newspaper accounts of people acting impulsively, behaving out of character, or even becoming suicidal while on antidepressants. There's still a lot of controversy over these reports, but I personally believe that some people, at least, are at risk for increased stimulation or "overactivation," particularly if there is a family history of bipolar illness or if the patient is prone to mood cycle or irritability.

The risk of such side effects was disturbing enough. But, I told Sarah, medication posed even more troubling concerns, particularly for a young person like her, who would most likely be facing a tendency to depression for the rest of her life.

SSRIS: BLOCKING THE REUPTAKE PUMP

My concern was rooted in the very nature of antidepressants. Let's start with a closer look at SSRIs, the most commonly prescribed class of antidepressants, and the type of medication that would have been appropriate for Sarah.

Like most antidepressants, SSRIs work in a way that tends to be self-limiting. They're often very effective in the short term while frequently losing their effectiveness in the long term. In fact, if patients don't change their diet and lifestyle while taking SSRIs, this medication can in some cases leave them even worse off than they were before.

Sarah had observed this very phenomenon with her mother. Like so many patients who are given medications with no nutritional or lifestyle support, Sarah's mother had gotten into a downward spiral in which medications both worsened her problem and grew less effective in treating it.

The problem with SSRIs lies in the way they operate to improve mood and energy. As the name implies, these selective serotonin reuptake inhibitors *selectively inhibit* the *reuptake* of *serotonin;* in plain English, they block the reuse of serotonin within the brain. As we saw in Chapter 2, serotonin is a brain chemical that is basic to our sense of calm, self-confidence, and well-being. It circulates through our brain as it is released from one nerve cell, moves across the synapse, and fits into the receptor of the next neuron. That moment of reception triggers a response in the neuron, and if the response is repeated often enough, we start to feel good. That's why higher levels of serotonin floating in the synaptic fluid—the fluid between nerve cells—are a sure-fire antidote to depression, listlessness, low self-esteem, and anxiety. As our neurons begin to respond to the serotonin, our mood improves, we become energized, and we even start feeling better about ourselves.

As we also saw in Chapter 2, the luckiest people among us are born with naturally high levels of serotonin. For some reason, these happy people seem to be able to manufacture enough serotonin to keep their synapses flooded with the chemical, and so "their tank is always full"— that is, their neurons have a constant supply of this "feel-good" chemical.

On the other hand, people who have undergone significant amounts of stress, had stressful childhoods, or possess a genetic tendency to depression all struggle with short- or long-term serotonin shortages. Their neurons aren't getting the serotonin they need—and depression is the result.

What happens to serotonin after the neuron receives it? As soon as the initial connection is made—producing the happy response I just described—the cell releases its serotonin molecule back into the synapse. And if the serotonin remains in the synaptic fluid, various brain chemicals break it down and eliminate it from the body. Eventually, the body has to make more serotonin, or depression will recur.

There's an intermediate step, though, between using serotonin the first time and expelling it from our brains. To avoid having to continually manufacture new serotonin, our efficient brains have found a way to recycle that vital chemical. A "reuptake pump" captures the serotonin molecule as soon as it is released from the receiving neuron and brings the chemical right back into the cell that just released it. There it is stored, and eventually, released again.

SSRIs work by blocking that pump, preventing the reuptake and re-cycling of serotonin molecules. As a result, serotonin stays in our synapses longer. For people with low serotonin levels, whose receptor neurons are used to chasing every scarce molecule of the "feel-good fluid," SSRIs create a whole new experience. Suddenly it seems as though the receptor neurons are being flooded with this soothing chem-ical. Instead of scrambling for a few serotonin molecules, they can luxu-riate in what seems like a new abundance.

As a result, people on SSRIs often feel terrific when they first start taking the meds. Their sense of well-being improves, their mood lifts, and their depression seems to dissipate. Many people describe this expe-rience as a veil or a cloud being lifted from their brains. People who have been depressed for years say that they finally know how "normal" people feel. These once-depressed patients may still have ups and downs, but they feel that their moods are within bounds. Instead of creeping along the edge of an abyss, they're merely strolling along a somewhat uneven path—sometimes uphill, sometimes downhill, but never with the sense of dread and doom they used to experience every day.

For the first few weeks or even months, these newly medicated pa-tients continue to improve. Now that they feel more resilient, they're better able to handle the curveballs that life throws their way. A minor setback—like Jennifer's lonely feeling when her roommate went off without her—seems truly minor instead of a trigger for overwhelming sorrow. "I finally get what people mean by 'don't sweat the small stuff,'" one of my patients once told me. "Before, I never even knew there *was* small stuff."

As I observe patients who begin taking SSRIs, I'm always struck by how many areas of their lives improve. They tend to feel better about themselves, less worthless, more hopeful and confident. The negative self-talk ("I never do anything right," "Who'd want to be *my* friend?," "No wonder no one likes me") diminishes, often to be replaced by the tentative beginnings of positive self-talk ("I'm learning every day," "I'd make a great friend," "Actually, a lot of people do like me"). They can enjoy themselves more, are better able to concentrate, and can be more productive. I've seen many of my patients become more extroverted, better able to put themselves out into the world. They also become braver, more able to take chances—and to pick themselves up and start over again when their chances don't work out.

Who wouldn't want to feel that way? If there were indeed a pill that could produce that effect, why shouldn't I prescribe it to Sarah?

"The Medication Doesn't Work Anymore"

As you may have guessed from my description, the problem with SSRIs is that often their effect is only temporary. By preventing the reuptake pump from recycling serotonin, the brain experiences the temporary high of an increased serotonin level. But remember: The body isn't actually producing more serotonin. It's only retaining the existing serotonin in the synapses for a longer time. Sooner or later, a new stressor is likely to come along and deplete the brain's already low supply of serotonin. Or perhaps you live such a stressful life that your serotonin stores are being gradually depleted all the time. Medication doesn't replenish your serotonin levels—it only manipulates them. So if you haven't done anything to boost your serotonin levels, either ongoing stress or some new problem will most likely drive your serotonin stores down to depressive levels once again.

Of course some people take SSRIs only to counter a temporary setback—a particularly stressful period or sorrowful event. People who are normally free from depression can use the temporary uplift of the SSRIs to overcome a short-term crisis. So if you haven't suffered from depression before, or if you're only prone to it in response to acute stress, you can probably go on to live without your medication, confident that your body is once again prepared to make all the serotonin you need.

But if, like Sarah and her mother, you have spent a lifetime struggling with depression, you've probably never been an efficient producer or manager of this soothing chemical. So unless you've done something to boost your serotonin production—starting a serotonin-friendly diet (Chapter 4), taking nutritional supplements (Chapter 5), undertaking healthy exercise and daily routines (Chapter 6), and practicing mindfulness (Step Three)—your serotonin levels are likely to remain low, and your risk of depression will remain high.

Unfortunately, most doctors and psychiatrists are unaware of the need to support serotonin production through these supplementary means. So usually, when a patient reports the return of depression, the doctor simply increases the dosage. The patient feels good—until once again, the brain exhausts the new supply. The cycle continues with the period of relief becoming shorter and shorter, until finally the dose becomes too high for the patient to tolerate or the medication simply becomes ineffective. Then the physician is likely to prescribe a new medication, or to combine two medications, and the cycle begins all over again. This was the pattern Sarah had observed with her mother. No wonder it scared her.

"I Wish I Could Get Off My Medication"

It's bad enough when SSRIs provide only short-term relief for depression, leaving patients right back where they started. But in some cases, SSRIs can make a patient's condition even worse.

Sarah, for example, had spent a lifetime struggling with low levels of serotonin. As a result, her brain had become very efficient at using any serotonin that was available. To compensate for the scarcity of serotonin molecules in the synaptic fluid, each of Sarah's nerve cells had developed numerous serotonin receptors—the portion of the cell designed to receive serotonin—and those receptors had become highly sensitive and adept. It was as though, if even a single serotonin molecule floated by, a thousand receptive hands immediately reached out to snatch it. This process of heightening one's sensitivity is known as "up-regulation."

So far, so good. Although Sarah isn't as happy and energetic as she would like, she has at least adapted to her condition. She has achieved what biologists call a state of *homeostasis*, in which an organism has become used to the way things are and resists any effort to change.

If Sarah were to start taking SSRIs, though, her situation would change dramatically. Although her serotonin levels wouldn't be any higher than they ever were, her receiving neurons would feel as if they are. So as the nerve cells happily soak up the new serotonin, they gradually reduce the number and sensitivity of their receptors. After all, with so much serotonin around, why work so hard at capturing and using it? Instead of a thousand eager hands snatching at a single scarce molecule, it's as though only a few hands reach out lazily to scoop up the new abundance. This process of decreasing sensitivity is known as "down-regulation."

Remember, Sarah's serotonin levels are still fairly low—but now her nerve cells have lost their heightened ability to make use of the scarce substance. So what happens if her serotonin levels drop even further, in response to a new stress? Those few lazy hands reaching out for serotonin will discover a new scarcity that they're not equipped to deal with. Sarah will be even less able to respond to stress than she was before—and even more in need of medication.

Likewise, if Sarah tries to stop her medication without having done anything to raise her serotonin levels, what is likely to happen? Once again, she's struggling with low levels of the crucial chemical, but without the increased sensitivity and efficiency she had developed before she started taking the meds. Those thousand eager hands—the increased number of sensitive neuron receptors—have disappeared, replaced by fewer and less sensitive receptors. So Sarah's ability to withstand stressors will markedly decrease, her resiliency will drop to an even lower degree than before, and her vulnerability to depression will become even greater. As a result, she's likely to feel that she *needs* the medication. In effect, even though antidepressants are not technically habit-forming, Sarah—like her mother—could become dependent on them, unable to function without them despite their decreasing effectiveness and painful side effects.

Withdrawal Symptoms

Knowing how SSRIs work helps us understand why going off such meds quickly often produces withdrawal symptoms after even a single day of missed medications. Withdrawal usually reaches its peak within three to five days of suddenly stopping or lowering dosage, with such symptoms as mild headache, nausea, tingling sensations, seeing flashing lights, restlessness, insomnia, and irritability. Still more troubling is the so-called rebound effect of increased anxiety and depression, experienced at a level of severity even worse than before the meds were started. Often, patients are able to return to normal after this initially stressful period, but they may need weeks to recover, and sometimes the increased severity of anxiety and depression is overwhelming. Therefore, *do not attempt to stop taking antidepressants, or even to lower your dosage, without the supervision of an experienced primary-care doctor or psychiatrist.*

"There's Got to Be an Alternative"

I explained this basic biochemistry to Sarah, who found it comforting to finally understand the cycle of serotonin depletion that had plagued her mother. I also pointed out that if Sarah didn't take immediate steps to respond to her own depression, it was likely to get worse. At this point, she still had a choice. In a few months, her symptoms might have worsened to the point where medication would indeed be her best option.

"Of course," I told her, "the pills are always there as a backup. But in your case, the symptoms are still mild enough that you could probably give more natural measures a try."

Sarah took a deep breath. "If there's even a chance that those other options would work," she answered, "I'd like to start with them."

We agreed that Sarah would begin a short course of psychotherapy with one of my colleagues, start getting regular exercise, change her diet to the serotonin-enhancing regime I describe in the next chapter, and begin taking B vitamins and fish-oil supplements (see Chapter 5). During more stressful times, I suggested that she add a dosage of 5-HTP, a supplement that helps the brain produce serotonin (again, see Chapter 5). If she didn't respond to these measures, Sarah agreed, she would come back to see me so we could discuss our next move.

Sarah was excited to have options presented to her that involved more natural ways to replenish her brain and gave her a greater measure of control over her own health. She left feeling hopeful for the first time in months, and it was obvious that her mood had improved just in the time we had spent together. I saw her again several weeks later to check on her progress, and her symptoms had improved markedly. While she still had some occasional down times, she no longer worried about them or saw them as a harbinger of a downward spiral. She now saw them as a simple sign of stress overload or some other temporary cause of imbalance, and was able to take immediate steps to replenish herself.

Sarah was particularly relieved not to have gone on medication. "Maybe at some point I will need to take antidepressants for a while," she told me. "But whether that happens or not, I don't have to end up like my mother. I can overcome the depression, with or without medications. And I don't have to stay on medications forever—it can be a temporary thing."

Although we've focused so far on SSRIs and serotonin depletion, the principle is the same with other types of antidepressants. Other medications do the same thing for norepinephrine and dopamine that SSRIs do for serotonin: They manipulate brain chemistry but don't restore it. And you may run into the same problems with them as with the SSRIs if you don't do enough to remedy the cause of the depletion.

EVALUATING YOUR NEED FOR MEDICATION

Although I encouraged Sarah to try alternatives to antidepressants, I want to make one thing perfectly clear: No one should look upon the need for medication as a failure or a sign of weakness. Over the years, I've seen many, many examples of how antidepressants have made an extraordinary difference in the lives of my patients, enabling people who had lived "under a cloud" for years to come out into the sunshine and enjoy their lives, or empowering people who'd had a lifelong history of feeling timid and worthless to discover their strengths and their worth. I believe too deeply in the profound interconnection of mind and body ever to think that depression is "all in your mind" or that it can simply be willed away. Nor do I believe that diet, exercise, meditation, and the other techniques described in this book are always sufficient, or that they work equally well for everyone. Sometimes, whether for a few months or as a lifelong support, medications are simply needed, and we should all be grateful that they work as well as they do.

However, whether or not you are on medications, I also believe that if you're suffering from any type of depression, you need to consider how to nourish your brain with the right type of diet, supplements, and exercise, and how to feed your soul with the meditations and heart-opening techniques that are right for you. So I hope you'll see this chapter as one end of a spectrum of choices, opening up new choices rather than precluding any one approach.

How do you know if you do need medications? In the end, this is a decision you must make with your doctor, therapist, or health professional, based on the specifics of your situation and the particular way your own biochemistry responds to stress, nutrition, exercise, and other types of therapy. Here, however, are a few guidelines to help you evaluate your condition:

You might consider short-term medication if . . .

. . . you have undergone one or more severe stressors—a death in the family, a move, a job loss or job change, the birth of a child, or some other life-altering event—and are unable to "bounce back" after more than a month.

. . . you are finding yourself unable to function normally in your daily life.

. . . you have lost the zest for life, finding it hard to get interested in things or to experience pleasure in them.

. . . you have recently had periods of prolonged, unexplained sadness that last for more than a few hours at a time and occur more than once a week.

. . . sleep, appetite and sexual interest are diminished.

. . . you are plagued by suicidal or self-destructive thoughts.

You might consider long-term medication if . . .

. . . you have had frequent or prolonged periods of being unable to function.

. . . you have had frequent or prolonged periods of unexplained sadness over the past several years.

. . . you are subject to frequent or periodic bouts of disabling depression or anxiety that interfere with your ability to work, socialize, or enjoy your life.

. . . you have a family history of depression, alcoholism, or suicide.

. . . you have a long history of suicidal thoughts.

. . . you have already had one or more depressive episodes of such an extent that you experienced devastating consequences.

4

FEED YOUR BRAIN

Mary had been depressed since her early twenties, including a few severe episodes in which she'd stayed in bed for two or three weeks at a time, unable even to get dressed or perform basic household tasks. As she'd approached menopause, her depression had worsened, and now, in her early fifties, she had been taking Paxil, an SSRI, for three years. Mary had always struggled a bit with her weight, but by the time she came to me, she had gained twenty-five pounds and was in despair.

"I don't know whether it's my hormones, the Paxil, or the way this depression gets me down," she told me. I could see that she was trying to put a happy face on things, but beneath the surface cheerfulness, her voice sounded tired and discouraged. "I just don't seem to have any energy anymore, and so of course, I don't exercise. I feel like a big whale just beached up on the shore somewhere."

Although Mary had supposedly come to me for help with her depression, I could see that her weight was almost as pressing a concern. "I just don't know how I got this heavy," she kept repeating. The more we talked, the clearer it became that Mary's weight gain was integrally bound up in her feelings of hopelessness, worthlessness, and despair. "I know I don't have any willpower," she said once. Another time she remarked, "I *should* be able to stop eating so much, but somehow I just don't."

Mary's sense of failure, and her increased sense of helplessness about being able to change her life, were clearly making her depression worse. And, as she talked on, I could see that her depression was contributing to her weight gain as well. "I get to feeling so low, and then I just *eat*," she told me. "Sometimes it seems like food is the only thing that cheers me up."

DIET, DEPRESSION, AND YOUR BRAIN CHEMISTRY

Mary was struggling with a problem that many of my patients encounter: the close connection between food choices, weight, depression, and brain chemistry. And, like many of my patients, she was caught in a vicious cycle. The choices she was making led her to feel worse—and the worse she felt, the harder it was for her to make healthy choices.

The good news, though, for Mary and for you, is that diet can have a revolutionary effect on your brain chemistry. Once you know what you need to eat, you can feel markedly better almost immediately, simply by cutting out a few unhealthy choices and adding the foods for which your brain and body are literally starving. It can be hard to make the switch, at first, especially when you're feeling low. The thought of giving up that sack of chips while you watch TV or of switching from pasta to brown rice might seem to be a terrible bereavement, the loss of one of your few reliable pleasures. But I promise you, if you're willing to try the suggestions in this chapter, you'll experience an almost instantaneous improvement in your mood. You'll almost certainly feel more energized and healthy—and you'll probably lose some weight.

One word of warning: All of us tend to be emotional about our food choices, and it can be hard to hear someone suggest any changes, particularly when we're feeling low. So if you find that reading this chapter—or just thinking about reading this chapter—makes you anxious, sad, or fearful, take a deep breath, remind yourself that you're allowed to make changes at your own pace, and keep reading. You really can eat your way into a better mood—and your brain will start rewarding you as soon as you do.

WEIGHT, SUGAR, AND DEPRESSION

For Mary, as for many depressed people, weight and depression were interconnected. Although it's too simple to say either that weight gain leads to depression or that depression causes obesity, there are many ways in which being overweight and being depressed reinforce each other.

First, many people, like Mary, find it soothing to eat, and often turn to food when they're stressed, upset, or anxious. And the foods to which they turn tend to be high in sugar (candy, ice cream, pastries, sodas) and in refined carbs (potatoes, bread, pasta, crackers, chips, and other foods made with white flour), both of which raise the blood sugar very quickly. Indeed, Mary told me that when she felt lonely, sad, or anxious, she liked to fill up on sweet and starchy foods, which seemed, at least temporarily, to have a cheering effect.

I explained to Mary that this temporary relief from anxiety or sadness was not a purely psychological phenomenon. She was probably suffering from a beta-endorphin deficiency on top of a serotonin-deficient depression.

Beta-endorphins are another type of neurotransmitter. Like serotonin, they also help create a sense of well-being, not so much by soothing us as by boosting our feelings of self-esteem, connectedness to others, and emotional stability. They help us tolerate pain—both physical and emotional—and they also seem to be involved in our ability to take personal responsibility for our actions.

Sugar—along with alcohol, heroin, morphine, and other pain medications known as *opiates*—stimulates the release of these vital chemicals, at least for a short time. As a result, we often crave sugar when we're low on beta-endorphins, in an unconscious attempt to rebalance our brain chemistry. Other symptoms of beta-endorphin depression include low tolerance of pain; feeling tearful and reactive; low self-esteem; feeling overwhelmed by others' pain; feeling isolated, depressed, and hopeless; thinking like a victim; and feeling emotionally overwhelmed.

So, I told Mary, when she ate sweet and starchy foods, she triggered a release of beta-endorphin molecules, temporarily boosting her b-e levels and soothing her emotional pain. But hitting her body with this sudden influx of "feel-good" chemicals caused her body to metabolize the chemical even more quickly. Thus Mary's momentary beta-endorphin "high" was followed by a longer-lasting "low"—which in turn set off a new craving for sugar or starch.

As a result, the more often Mary ate sweet or starchy foods, the more intensely she craved them. She had inadvertently created a near-addictive situation in which she literally needed high-sugar, high-carb foods to balance her brain chemistry—even though this type of food was guaranteed to keep her off balance.

Sugar Cravings: Not Just in Your Mind

Animal studies confirm that the relief some of us get from eating sugar isn't just psychological—it's an actual brain-chemistry reaction. In one experiment, Blass and colleagues studied two groups of baby mice who were separated from their mothers and left alone for six minutes. Their resulting "isolation distress" was considered to be a kind of animal equivalent to our own human version of depression. The depressed mice who were given sugar water cried only seventy-five times during their isolation—as compared to the more than three hundred cries that came from the mice left alone with no sweet treat to alleviate their emotional pain. Apparently, the young mice were literally "medicating" their depression with sugar.

Why did sugar have this remarkable effect? Researchers thought that perhaps the sweet food stimulated the release of extra beta-endorphin molecules. Since b-e's help us cope with physical and emotional pain, the sugar had a literally soothing effect. Researchers confirmed their theory by giving both groups of mice Naltrexone, a drug that blocks beta-endorphin receptors. If you take Naltrexone, it doesn't matter how many beta-endorphins you release—you won't get any relief from pain. Sure enough, when the sugar-fed mice were given Naltrexone, they lost all interest in the sweet substance, suggesting that their only reason for their sweet tooth had been to stimulate the release of beta-endorphins.

Numbed by Naltrexone, both groups of mice cried equally often. The poor baby mice were still depressed—but now even sugar couldn't make them feel better.[1]

Frankly, if eating sweet foods had no other effects, I'd probably counsel all my patients to self-medicate with them. Unfortunately, sugar is terrifically bad for your health, causing weight gain and associated with cancer, heart disease, and a host of other disorders. Moreover, the kind of relief you get from eating sweet and starchy foods is by its very nature short-lived and problematic. Yes, the sugar sets off a temporary release of beta-endorphins that makes you feel better for a while. But your relief is soon erased by the crash that comes when your body metabolizes the beta-endorphins too quickly. The result is a sugar-addicted cycle that actively interferes with the long-term well-being you're really looking for. I do want to help you release more beta-endorphins—but in a slower, more steady way, through healthy diet, vigorous exercise, and the mental/spiritual approaches I explain in Step Three. I want you to enjoy long-term high levels of this feel-good chemical, rather than having you ride the emotional roller coaster induced by refined carbs and processed sugar.

Meanwhile, as I told Mary, every time you reach for a sweet dessert or starchy snack, you're actually trying to medicate your depression. So although I'd like you to switch to other foods, you shouldn't wonder that it's so difficult to do so—or to lose weight. You're not greedy, undisciplined, or out of control (although it may feel as if you are). You're simply responding to a very real biological problem.

ARE YOU SUGAR-SENSITIVE?

People with frequent or intense sugar/carb cravings, as well as people who respond strongly to refined sugar and starchy foods, suffer from a condition known as *sugar sensitivity,* a term coined by researcher Kathleen DesMaisons and discussed in her book *Potatoes Not Prozac.*[2] Although diet books often talk in terms of willpower or "making healthy choices," sugar-sensitive people may be genetically predisposed to both sugar craving and other addictions by having naturally low beta-endorphin levels. Their response to sweet foods (and narcotics) is thus exaggerated. Eating something sweet tends to send their blood sugar levels shooting sky-high, producing a corresponding rush of insulin. The insulin—released in extra-large doses to respond to the sugar spike—tends to overdo its job, with a correspondingly oversized drop in blood-sugar levels. Symptoms like dizziness, mental fog, irritability, or headaches are common along the way, as is a more or less constant state of stress as the body copes with too many extremes in too short a time. This stress in turn induces the adrenal glands to release excess amounts of stress hormones, exhausting the adrenal glands from their continual use. The result is often fatigue and—yet again—depression.

Like many aspects of nutrition, sugar sensitivity is a spectrum rather than a clearly identifiable condition. Some people may be highly sensitive to sugar, while others have milder versions of this condition. Depending on your diet, lifestyle, and emotional state, you may experience greater or lesser degrees of sugar sensitivity over your lifetime. Women in particular often become more or less sensitive to sugar at various times in their menstrual cycle or in response to menopause or menarche (the onset of menstruation). Some people become sugar-sensitive only or primarily in response to stress; others are sugar-sensitive all the time. As a result, there's no one test for this condition, and many conventional doctors are rather skeptical about it. From my observation and clinical practice, however, I believe sugar sensitivity is an important factor in weight gain as well as depression.

If you are sugar-sensitive, your strategy should be a slow but steady elimination of foods containing processed sugar and refined carbs, even as you gradually add complex carbs into your diet. You probably shouldn't get off sugar "cold turkey," but you should make a concerted effort to switch from processed sugar to complex carbs. You'll be amazed at how much better you feel in the long run.

FAST FOOD FOR THE BRAIN: COMPLEX VS. REFINED CARBS

Even if you're not sugar-sensitive, you should take the advice I just gave, which will have enormous benefits for your mood, energy, and overall health: *switch from refined to complex carbohydrates*. Refined carbohydrates include processed sugar, honey, white rice, and products made with white flour, including breads, pastas, crackers, cookies, and pastries. Complex carbs include legumes, starchy vegetables, and whole grains. Your brain desperately needs complex carbs to function, while refined carbohydrates tend to throw you off balance. So anytime you're struggling with mood, energy, or depression, cut back on the refined carbs or cut them out entirely, even as you up your intake of complex carbohydrates.

Let's take a closer look at what carbohydrates are and why your brain needs them—in the right form. Carbohydrates, also known as starches, provide fuel for the brain and the rest of your body. As you consume a chickpea stew, a bag of corn chips, or a big bowl of ice cream, your body metabolizes the carbohydrates contained in the food and converts them into *glucose*, or blood sugar. When your blood sugar levels are low, you feel hungry, and sometimes you experience a number of other symptoms as well—fatigue, dizziness, mental fog, irritability, and for some people, headache. When your blood-sugar levels are high, on the other hand, you feel full, energized, alert, and able to function at peak efficiency. And if your blood-sugar levels are *too* high, such as after you gobble down a candy bar or quickly drink a large soda, you might get a "sugar rush"—the feeling of being revved up, agitated, or overly stimulated.

As you can see, blood-sugar levels are crucial to energy, functioning, and mood. But not all carbohydrates affect our blood sugar in the same way. Refined carbohydrates are already broken down, leaving the body little work in order to turn them into blood sugar. As a result, they tend to send blood-sugar levels skyrocketing—that quick rush we know so well—often followed by a crash that leaves us craving another fix, more sweet and starchy foods to boost our blood sugar once again.

The more quickly a food is converted into glucose, the more rapid are its effects—and the less time they last. That's why a refined carb—like a candy bar or some fruit juice—gives you a quick lift. It's also why, soon after you've consumed it, you experience an equally quick drop in energy, efficiency, and mood. The sudden influx of glucose triggers an equally sudden rush of insulin, the hormone your body uses to break down blood sugar. For many people, the "low" that follows a sugar rush is even lower than where they were before, creating yet another craving for something sweet.

Complex or unrefined carbohydrates, by contrast, are not yet processed. They contain a tough substance called fiber, which slows down the process of metabolizing these foods. You'll never get a sugar rush from complex carbs—your body has to work too hard and too long to convert them into sugar. As a result, these foods offer a slow, steady release of glucose into your system, a much more stable way of feeling full, alert, and energized.

You can see why complex carbs are so much better for your moods. They're also better for your brain, which much prefers to get a relatively constant supply of glucose. So switching from refined to complex carbs will immediately help you to feel calmer, "fuller," and more in control of your appetite—especially if you're sugar-sensitive.

The Glycemic Index

You may have heard of something called the glycemic index, which is one attempt to measure the speed at which various carbohydrates are converted into blood sugar. This index forms the basis of some of the currently popular low-carb diets and is cited by many people as the key to making good dietary choices.

I'm a bit skeptical myself: A serving of carrots actually has a higher glycemic index than a candy bar, yet clearly carrots are a healthier choice. In my opinion, you don't need to worry too much about the glycemic index if you just keep in mind the difference between complex and refined carbs, and make the switch accordingly.

THE FAT FACTOR

Another key problem with Mary's diet was her excess consumption of unhealthy fats and her underconsumption of healthy ones. When I tell my depressed patients that certain fats are an essential component in their "healthy brain" diets, they often stare at me in surprise. By now, most of us realize that fats provide a much more concentrated source of calories than any other food source (nine calories per gram of fat compared to four calories per gram in proteins or carbs). This high-calorie infusion was crucial for the survival of our ancestors, who often had to go for long periods without food and needed to store their calories in the form of body fat. Now that obesity is a greater danger than starvation to most Americans, fat has become a dietary evil in many people's minds.

Certainly Mary had always viewed fat as "the enemy," though she confessed that she found it hard to resist the high-fat chips and french fries she often craved. Mary had also noticed that fat wasn't always beneficial to her mood. I often have to remind my patients that too much fat in a meal can leave you feeling sluggish, lethargic, and unhappy, especially if eaten in the middle of the day. Moreover, the wrong kinds of fats—hydrogenated fats and trans-fatty acids, found in margarine and processed foods—have been associated with numerous health problems, including cardiovascular disease, hypertension, and stroke.

But our bodies and brains need some fat to function—and the right kinds of fat contain elements that are crucial to overcoming depression. Moreover, extremely low levels of overall cholesterol—below 160—are associated with both depression and a higher risk of suicide, while cholesterol in adequate amounts helps boost the serotonin available within the synaptic fluid.[3] Cholesterol also helps us produce the neurotransmitters—including serotonin, norepinephrine, dopamine, and beta-endorphins—that our brains need to function: It's cholesterol that helps transport the proteins from which our brains make these vital chemicals. Finally, several key vitamins can be absorbed only in fat, so a fat deficiency can lead to a vitamin shortage—even if we're taking supplements.

Just as our body needs essential amino acids, so does it need the so-called *essential fatty acids* (EFAs)—the food elements that our body can't manufacture from other fats. The EFAs are the building blocks for nerve cells, and without them, the neurotransmitters and their receptors can't function properly.

Yet many people—particularly those suffering from depression—are omitting these crucial substances from their diets. So here's my second piece of simple advice: **If you're feeling depressed, boost your intake of essential fatty acids.** You may well need to cut back on the chips and fries. That doesn't mean you're getting enough fatty fish, fish oil, flaxseed oil, olive oil, nuts, and seeds—all of which you need to fight depression.

THOSE AMAZING OMEGAS

EFAs come in two major categories: Omega-3s and Omega-6s. Omega-3s are found in fatty or cold-water fish (salmon, bluefish, tuna, and halibut, among others) as well as some northern grains and nuts (including flax, canola, and walnuts). They seem to offer numerous health benefits, including lower cholesterol and triglyceride levels, lower blood pressure, joint lubrication, protection against inflammation, and support for the immune system—and possibly, reduction of depression.

Omega-6 fatty acids are found in plant-seed oils (flax, evening primrose, black currant, and borage), polyunsaturated vegetable oils (safflower, sunflower, corn, and soybean oils), and animal products, especially egg yolks and organ meats. Generally, Omega-6s are important for bodily growth, maintenance of skin and hair, regulating metabolism, reproductive activity, and the absorption and retention of calcium, and to help prevent heart disease, cancer, stroke, diabetes, and rheumatoid arthritis.

Changes in our modern diet may have contributed to a relative increase in consumption of Omega-6 fatty acids and a corresponding decrease in Omega-3s. Generally speaking, Omega-3 acids reduce inflammation, while Omega-6s promote it. Inflammation affects all organs, including the brain, and is suspected as one of the key causes of Alzheimer's disease and other causes of cognitive decline. So clearly, it would benefit your brain's and your body's health if you boost your Omega-3 intake and lower your consumption of Omega-6s.

Mary and I discussed her dietary choices at length. I told her that to overcome her depression and to boost her health in general, she needed to get at least half her fat calories from EFAs, making a determined effort to include more Omega-3s and fewer Omega-6s. Reorganizing her fat intake would not only improve Mary's mood and mental clarity, I told her. It would probably also help her lose weight, which would have additional benefits in helping her to overcome depression.

ANTIDEPRESSANTS AND WEIGHT GAIN

Mary faced one final obstacle in her efforts to lose weight and overcome depression—antidepressants. Unfortunately, medication intended to combat depression, while helpful in improving mood and energy, can also make it harder to lose weight.

The connections between antidepressants and weight gain are complex. For one thing, medications often increase appetite, making it harder for some people to resist high-calorie foods. At the same time, antidepressants also seem to affect blood-sugar metabolism and insulin function. While we don't fully understand the relationship between these processes and weight gain, we do know that as a result of their complex interactions, even people who reduce their calorie intake may find it hard to lose weight while on antidepressants.

MARY'S STRUGGLE WITH WEIGHT AND DEPRESSION

To develop a healthier eating plan for Mary, we began by reviewing her current eating habits. She told me that she usually either skipped breakfast or relied on a starchy start to her day, such as toast or a bagel. In her efforts to avoid calories, she'd eat a large salad for lunch. She'd save her biggest meal for dinner, which she thought should ideally include chicken or fish along with a vegetable and starch of some sort.

Indeed, most days, Mary would succeed in sticking to this regime—until later in the evening. Then she would binge on starchy snacks and sweet junk foods. No matter how guilty and ashamed she felt when she was done, she saw herself as powerless to stop the cycle.

The first thing I told Mary was that her attempts to limit calories early in the day might actually make it harder for her to resist binging later on. Starting the day with a starchy breakfast set her up for sugar and carb cravings that built in intensity until she finally satisfied them at the end of the evening. And depriving herself of protein until dinner not only made her more vulnerable to those cravings, it also kept her foggy, low energy, and prone to blood-sugar fluctuations. Eating good sources of protein throughout the day, on the other hand, would keep her energetic and alert, besides helping to stabilize her blood sugar.

Ultimately, Mary's emergence from depression involved several factors and required a great deal of support. After all, changing lifelong habits is no easy matter. She joined Weight Watchers for the group support, and also worked with a dietician well versed in the serotonin–food connection. (Although Mary seemed to have a beta-endorphin deficiency, she also suffered from serotonin depletion, which further intensified her depression and probably made it harder for her to lose weight as well.)

Mary began eating breakfasts that included fresh fruit (to satisfy her sugar cravings), high-fiber cereal (to provide the serotonin support she needed), and a good protein source like eggs, lean meat, or protein powder (to energize her for the day and help balance her blood sugar). She continued to have a salad at lunch, but now added a few ounces of chicken, tuna, or cottage cheese for protein (again, to boost her energy, balance her blood sugar, and combat her carbo cravings). She started eating a midafternoon snack of yogurt or a few nuts—both high in protein as well as rich in amino acids, which again helped her produce more serotonin—and finished the day with her usual well-balanced dinner. She felt as though she was eating a lot more than before, but this diet also helped her avoid her evening binges. Instead, she could get by with a small bedtime snack of a little cereal or a piece of whole-grain toast.

Mary didn't lose much weight at first, but she did start feeling better almost immediately. Increasing her protein while cutting back on the sugar and starch made her mentally clearer, stabilized her mood, and helped her get motivated. Her passion had always been artwork, and suddenly she found herself painting again. Although she remained on Paxil, she was able to reduce her medication almost immediately, with no drop in mood, most likely because her improved diet was enabling her to produce more serotonin and beta-endorphins. The drop in medication in turn helped her lose some weight more easily.

Suddenly Mary was feeling better about herself, with a tentative newfound faith in her ability to overcome this lifelong problem. Although Mary's severe history of depression meant that she might need to continue some form of medication for many years, we still both considered her a success story, as she'd cut her dose to less than half, was finally free of side effects, and felt better than she'd felt in twenty-five years.

Vitalizing Vitamins

Although your brain doesn't actually make serotonin, dopamine, and norepinephrine from vitamins and minerals, it needs these essential nutrients to enable their production process and to regulate their function. If you're eating a lot of highly processed or calorie-rich foods, you're probably not getting enough vitamins. Consider enhancing your daily diet with some of the supplements recommended in the next chapter. Better still, start boosting your vitamin intake by increasing your consumption of green, yellow, and leafy vegetables, such as broccoli, collard greens, spinach, and kale.

We're only just beginning to understand the role of vitamin and mineral shortages in depression, but here's a quick overview of some illuminating studies:

- *Folic acid:* A shortage of folic acid may be the most common vitamin deficiency in the world. If you're prone to depression, you'll want to be especially careful about consuming enough folic acid (also known as folate). Researchers in England found that one-third of the depressed patients they studied were deficient in this form of vitamin B—and that their conditions improved markedly when they were given supplements.[4] Good sources for folic acid include most dark green vegetables, including spinach, romaine lettuce, kale, and broccoli. Folic acid tends to disappear quickly, so it's best to eat these foods soon after they're picked, and to avoid overcooking.

- *Vitamin B_6:* A recent Harvard study of depressed patients found that at least one-quarter of them were not getting enough B_6.[5] You can raise your own B_6 quotient by eating meat, nuts, legumes, fish, bananas, and green leafy veggies.

- *Vitamin B_{12}:* A study published in the *American Journal of Psychiatry* in 2000 reported a clear correlation between depression and B_{12} deficiency—a correlation that was even stronger when depression was more severe.[6] You can find B_{12} in eggs, poultry, meat, shellfish, milk, and dairy products. Try eggs from flax-fed chickens, organic chicken, low-fat yogurt or cottage cheese, and skim milk.

A number of other studies suggest that minerals as well as vitamins may be crucial in balancing mood and improving the health of your brain. Because of the increasing use of chemicals and fertilizers in U.S. agriculture, vital minerals are being stripped from the soil, leading some researchers to express concern that we are generally not getting enough needed minerals in our diets, even if we're eating recommended amounts of fruits and vegetables.[7] So consider taking a mineral supplement or else eating more organic produce grown in mineral-rich soil.

EATING FOR MENTAL HEALTH

I know there's a lot of confusing information out there about diet and health. But what you eat can have such a revolutionary impact on how you feel that I strongly urge you to give the following "brain-healthy diet" a try, even if only for thirty days. I guarantee you'll feel so much better that you'll be motivated to eat well and feel better.

Your Brain-Healthy Diet: Eating for Improved Mental Health
- Eat fewer calories overall (unless you're seriously underweight).
- Restrict fats to 25 percent to 30 percent of your overall calories, and avoid eating large amounts of fats in the middle of the day, when they will slow you down, cloud your thinking, and set you up for fat cravings later on that night.
- Try to get most of your fat from healthy fat sources (olive oil, avocados) and essential fatty acids, such as fish oil, safflower oil, flax seed, borage or evening primrose oil, and nuts.
- Restrict your intake of refined sugar to 10 percent or less of your total calories. If you're sugar-sensitive, consider entirely eliminating sugar and refined carbohydrates (white rice and foods made from white flour, including most breads, pastas, and processed foods).
- Cut back to one or two cups per day of most caffeinated drinks—coffee, black tea, colas, chocolate drinks—and eliminate these drinks entirely if you suffer from anxiety, have trouble sleeping, or are prone to headache. You might substitute green tea for the other beverages, as it has very little caffeine and offers several other health benefits.
- Organize your diet around the following healthy foods:

   1. *Complex carbohydrates,* especially **whole grains** (rye and pumpernickel bread, oatmeal, barley, brown rice, millet, spelt, amaranth), beans and legumes (adzuki, black beans, pinto beans, lentils) and **root vegetables** (onions, turnips, rutabagas, carrots, sweet potatoes). **Three or more servings per day, four ounces per serving**
   2. *Lean protein,* especially **cold-water seafood, legumes,** and **soy products** (each of which has other health benefits as well). **Three servings per day, four to six ounces per serving**
   3. *Fresh fruits* (including at least one fruit per day that is high in vitamin C, such as a citrus fruit or a cup of fresh berries) and *dark green leafy vegetables* (don't overcook). **Five servings per day, one fruit or one-half cup vegetable per serving**

- Buy fresh, organic, seasonal, locally grown foods if you can afford them. They cost a bit more, but they're worth it. Not only do they taste better, but organic produce is far more nutritious than its commercial counterpart, and more likely to contain micronutrients—trace elements of minerals that remain in the soil when produce is farmed organically. Your body needs those minerals to facilitate neurotransmission—the process by which your brain sends messages to itself. In addition, organic foods have not been exposed to toxins, which stress your endocrine and immune systems (weakening your brain indirectly) while interfering with your central nervous system (weakening your brain directly).[8] Locally grown foods are more likely to be fresh, and eating them ensures that you get a wide variety of foods and nutrients.

- Drink plenty of pure water, at least six to eight glasses each day.
- Consider taking supplements, especially when your diet is poor, your stress levels are high, or you are suffering from depression (see Chapter 5).

Proteins: Building Blocks for the Brain

Protein is important for two reasons: It provides us with energy, and it supplies our brain with amino acids. These vital compounds are the building blocks of all the chemicals and tissues in our body, including those in the brain. For example, the amino acid *tryptophan*—found in turkey, dairy products, and nuts—is what the brain uses to make serotonin, while *phenylalanine* becomes norepinephrine, and *tyrosine* is used to make dopamine. Amino acids are found in high-protein foods, such as meats, dairy products, seafood, beans and legumes, and nuts.

Sometimes, our versatile bodies can actually convert one amino acid into another, compensating for a dietary shortage. But for several amino acids this conversion process is not possible, so they must be present in the diet. These are known as "essential amino acids," and I'm often struck at how many depressed patients are not getting enough of them. If you're suffering from or prone to depression, make sure you get enough daily protein, preferably in small, easily digested amounts that you consume throughout the day.

IF YOU SUFFER FROM A SEROTONIN SHORTAGE: EATING TO BOOST YOUR SEROTONIN LEVELS

People who are low in serotonin—whether over the short or the long term—should eat relatively more carbohydrates than other people, and they may not need quite as much protein. But if you're struggling to boost your serotonin production, you'll still need some quality protein throughout the day. In addition to protein's role in energy and muscle development, your brain also needs the amino acids contained in proteins to create serotonin, norepinephrine, and dopamine.

Tryptophan is the basic building block for serotonin. It's found in meats, dairy products, and nuts. However, tryptophan has trouble competing with the other amino acids found in proteins. That is, when you eat a high-protein meal, rich in several different types of amino acids, the other acids tend to shove tryptophan out of the way as the brain absorbs them first. That's why people low in serotonin need a diet rich in *complex carbohydrates*. As we saw earlier, the fiber in complex carbs requires the body to work harder and makes the whole digestion process take longer. Slowing down the digestive process allows tryptophan to "hang around" longer, giving it enough time to get into your neurons and causing serotonin levels to rise.

If you're a sugar-sensitive person, you're probably also low in serotonin, so it's especially important for you to replace sweet and starchy foods with complex carbs. Make the switch gradually, though. If you cut out the sweet things too quickly, you can actually go into a form of withdrawal after a few days or even a few weeks, experiencing somewhat milder versions of the symptoms you'd get from abruptly going off SSRIs or other serotogenic antidepressants. (For more on withdrawal symptoms, see Chapter 3.) If you've ever tried out a low-carb, high-protein diet, particularly one that restricts your carbs drastically for the first few weeks, you might have found yourself so moody and irritable that you just couldn't stay away from the sugar and starch, aggravating your original problem and most likely increasing your weight. So if you're a sugar-sensitive type, give yourself a few weeks to make the transition away from sugars. Eventually, you should cut out refined carbs almost completely while getting the largest percentage of your calories from complex carbs.

My Recommendations

- Eat a wide variety of complex carbs throughout the day:

  1. *Whole grains*, especially those that you cook, like brown rice, millet, barley, oats, amaranth. Don't rely solely on whole-wheat bread or cold cereals. Your body needs nutrients from a wide variety of foods.
  2. *Beans/legumes*, which are also good protein sources
  3. *Root vegetables*, such as potatoes, sweet potatoes, carrots, onions, rutabagas, and turnips; as well as *squash* and *pumpkins*

- Get enough protein throughout the day. If you're low in serotonin, I don't recommend a high-protein diet. But you do need at least some protein in each meal and most snacks.
- Eat plenty of fresh fruits and green, leafy vegetables. While these don't contain the elements used to manufacture serotonin, they do contain vitamins and minerals that the brain needs to undertake the production process.
- Eat a wide variety of nuts, which contain both essential fatty acids and a small amount of protein. Because of their concentrated fats, nuts are high in calories, so don't overdo—a small handful each day will suffice.
- Eat regularly. Never skip breakfast. Try to eat something every four to five hours that you are awake. Have a small midmorning and midafternoon snack, and try a pure complex-carbohydrate snack at bedtime. By the way, there is some evidence to suggest that people with *seasonal affective disorder* may find light therapy more effective if they eat a midafternoon carbo-rich snack. (For more on seasonal affective disorder, see Chapter 6.)
- Eat plenty of serotonin-enhancing foods. (See Appendix A.)

IF YOU SUFFER FROM A NOREPINEPHRINE/ DOPAMINE EXCESS: EATING TO LOWER YOUR NOREPI/DOPA LEVELS

I believe that people who suffer from an agitated depression—marked by feelings of anger, irritability, or excess energy—are responding to an imbalance that includes too little serotonin and too much norepi/dopa.

You should eat to boost your serotonin levels, as described above—but with one modification. Given the excessive amounts of dopamine and/or norepinephrine in your brain, you would do well to eat very small amounts of protein, at least until things calm down. Get plenty of healthy carbs and essential fatty acids into your diet, and avoid highly concentrated protein sources, especially meat and seafood. In fact, I'd suggest a good old-fashioned vegetarian diet, in which you eat a combination of beans and whole grains as your protein source, at least until you recover.

IF YOU SUFFER FROM A NOREPINEPHRINE/ DOPAMINE SHORTAGE: EATING TO BOOST YOUR NOREPI/DOPA LEVELS

In many ways, this is an easier task than eating for serotonin. The amino acids used to produce these energizing biochemicals are *tyrosine* for dopamine and *phenylalanine* for norepinephrine—amino acids readily found in all sorts of protein foods and more easily assimilated into the brain than is tryptophan. So if you're suffering from a norepi/dopa deficiency, your main goal is to eat enough high-quality proteins throughout the day and to combine your protein sources with other appropriate foods.

Most of us don't need to be as alert or energetic in the evening, when our bodies and brains want to calm down, preparing for bed and a deep sleep. So loading up on a high-protein meal only hours before the day is over is the worst possible timing, particularly if the high-protein dinner is preceded by a high-fat lunch. You're much better off with a high-protein breakfast and lunch, and a moderate-protein dinner, with a relatively low amount of fat at each meal. (If you must load up on fat, save it for evening, as it will probably make you tired and sluggish—not a pleasant feeling, but less of a problem in the evening than in the midst of your workday. And a high-fat breakfast or lunch can set up powerful fat cravings that persist throughout the day.)

Breaking your old patterns can be challenging, but you'll feel so much better, the change will seem worthwhile. As an added bonus, you'll probably lose some weight!

How Much Protein Do You Need?

Like almost every other important question, the answer to this one is, "It depends." Men usually need more protein than women, while people with more lean muscle mass need more protein than those with more fat. And of course, the more strenuous exercise you get, the more protein you need.

Here is an easy way to approximate your ideal protein serving. Look at the palm of your hand—not the fingers, just your palm. At each meal, your ideal protein serving should be roughly the same size, whether you're talking about chicken, beef, seafood, or tofu. For most women, that would be roughly three or four ounces, while for most men the serving size is about five or six ounces.

My Recommendations

- Eat moderate amounts of high-quality, low-fat proteins with every meal and snack.
- Eat relatively small amounts of complex carbohydrates, but again, consume these throughout the day. If you've got really sluggish energy, and especially if you've got a weight problem, you can probably get by with far fewer carb-based calories, and you should focus, of course, on complex carbs. Ideally, each carb serving would equal one to two times the size of your palm.
- Enjoy unlimited servings of salad greens and fresh vegetables. These healthy choices have very few calories and lots of vitamins and minerals. They're a great way to fill up and to get your system moving.
- Eat breakfast! Skipping breakfast is many people's Achilles' heel, and it's a particular problem of people who need to consume more protein. If you enjoy breakfast meats, try some lean ham or Canadian bacon, which has less fat than regular bacon. If, like so many of us, you don't have time to cook, consider one of the many good protein powders for your morning pick-me-up. (See the list of suggested protein powders, in Appendix B.) You can mix your powder into a glass of juice, or make a fruit smoothie with juice or milk plus fresh or frozen berries. If you're feeling adventurous, sardines, tuna, or other cold-water fish makes a great protein-rich start to your day. And, if you can, vary your protein sources—eggs one

morning, yogurt the next, protein powders on the third. The more variety, the more nutrients—and the less strain on your system.

- Enjoy your eggs. This nearly perfect food once had a bad rap as a dangerous source of cholesterol, but nutritionists now understand that eggs are actually good for your heart and circulation, especially if you get them from farm-raised free-range chickens, and even more so if you eat eggs from flax-fed chickens, which inserts some brain-healthy Omega-3 into your diet.
- Eat modest amounts of food often, at least three meals and two snacks daily. An average person needs four hundred to six hundred calories per meal and one hundred to two hundred calories per snack. To put this in perspective, one large order of fries at a fast-food restaurant has about six hundred calories—and so does a chicken stir-fry chock-full of vegetables, a flavorful sauce, and a bit of rice. Which do you think your brain would prefer?
- Eat light. Limit complex carbs, and reduce or eliminate refined carbs and unhealthy fats. Eat plenty of fresh fruits, vegetables, and salads. Think of how your body likes you to eat in the heat of summer—light, fresh foods with plenty of water content. Try to stay with those foods, especially if your energy drops noticeably during the winter.
- Go nuts! Eat a variety of nuts and seeds, choosing from the list in Appendix B. They are great sources of both protein and healthy fats, and a small handful of twelve to twenty nuts makes an ideal between-meal snack.
- Eat plenty of dopamine/norepinephrine–enhancing foods. (See Appendix B.)

How Brain-Healthy Is Your Weight Loss?: A Look at Current U.S. Diets

- *Atkins Diet.* This low-carb high-protein weight-loss plan starts out pretty harshly, with almost no calories from carbohydrates in the first several weeks of the diet. This sudden loss of carbs is fairly hard on most people and may be especially difficult for someone who is serotonin-deficient. Atkins is also a high-fat diet that pays little attention to the difference between healthy and unhealthy fats—again, a problem for someone who needs a certain level of healthy fats for optimum brain function. The goal of Atkins is to create a metabolic state called "ketosis," which may not be safe for everyone. And while many people do lose weight quickly in their early days on Atkins, they often experience a "rebound" with later weight gain that can easily exceed the initial weight. I personally would not recommend this diet for anyone who struggles with serotonin deficiency. Norepi/dopa–deficient dieters might do all right on the high protein levels, but other aspects of the plan are not necessarily beneficial for their overall health and weight.

- *The Zone.* This more moderate diet plan is also high in protein, but it's more careful to balance the fats, carbs, and protein, and there's no harsh initial phase. There is much to recommend in this balanced approach, in which you ideally get 30 percent of your calories from fat, 30 percent from protein, and 40 percent from carbohydrates, with an emphasis on the right kinds of fats and on complex, healthy carbs. And this diet suggests, as I do, three small meals and two snacks each day, spaced out over every four to five waking hours. For many people with weight or mood problems, this could be a good maintenance diet. But it can be rather hard to follow and I think it can feel a little compulsive to be so careful about getting just the right combination of calories and eating at just the right times. This diet also can be a somewhat difficult transition for someone with a serotonin deficiency.

- *South Beach Diet.* Similar in many ways to Atkins, I think this eating plan is a fairly substantial improvement. The initial low-carb phase is less extreme than Atkins, and there is much more emphasis on limiting fats, getting the right type of fat, and paying attention to complex vs. refined carbs. I also think that this diet is easier to maintain longer term. If you've got a norepi/dopa–deficient depression, you might do very well on South Beach. If you're serotonin-deficient, however, it might be hard for you to cut back on the carbs so quickly.

- *Fat Flush Plan.* This is the only popular diet I know of that addresses the question of toxicity, the dangers to our systems that come from a rapid loss of weight. Because we store pesticides, artificial hormones, preservatives, and other toxins in our fat cells, losing weight quickly can expose us to these poisons too suddenly unless we are detoxing at the same time we're slimming down. I like the idea of attending not only to calories and weight loss but also to cleansing and detox, and there are many foods on this diet that I consider "serotonin-friendly." Still, the primary purpose of this diet is not to improve mood, and I think that, for most people dealing with depression, a more gradual transformation of diet may be more helpful than the sudden changes that the Fat Flush plan recommends.

- *Weight Watchers, Jenny Craig, and other weight-loss groups.* These organizations usually help members watch food choices and calories, which can be very helpful for weight loss. I also strongly recommend the group support, which helps create community—something that has benefited even my patients who have not lost weight. Again, however, these approaches focus on weight loss rather than mood, with too little attention paid to healthy fats and complex carbs. Likewise, their packaged foods, while containing fewer calories, are not otherwise the healthiest choices available.

- *Eat Right For Your Type.* In the book describing this diet plan, Peter D'Adamo suggests that people do best by following a diet specific to their blood type (A, B, AB, and O), based on the theory that our prehistoric ancestors evolved under different conditions and so became suited to different diets. For example, Type-O people can supposedly trace their origins to hunter-gatherers, so they need a diet higher in meats, fish and poultry, nuts, seeds, and berries. They don't tolerate dairy or grains as well as the types whose ancestors were sedentary farmers (who should favor grains) or wanderers (who should favor dairy). This approach has been frequently criticized for sketchy science by skeptics who point out that blood types probably evolved from animals and that the research done by D'Adamo and his father is not widely accepted. However, I've seen many people swear by the good results they claim to have gotten from this way of eating, and I do like the notion that each of us needs our own diet—no single weight-loss or nutritional plan is right for everyone.

FOOD SENSITIVITIES

Over the past few decades, alternative and complementary physicians have stressed the concept of "food sensitivity" or "food intolerance," in which an otherwise healthy person has a poor reaction to certain types of foods, particularly wheat and other grains or dairy products. Food sensitivities are far subtler than true allergies, which tend to have far more obvious symptoms (diarrhea, hives, wheezing, and the like). Likewise, sensitivities are not the same as food addictions, in which eating a particular food gives short-term relief while producing symptoms later.

In food sensitivities, by contrast, the body reacts so subtly that we either don't pay attention or we don't associate the ill effect with having eaten something. So if you suffer from depression, I believe it's important for you to consider the possibility that some of your food choices may be affecting your mood by setting off such sensitivities.

Foods to which many people are sensitive include wheat, corn, coffee, sugar, dairy, eggs, beef, potatoes, pork, oranges, carrots, yeast, apples, chicken, lettuce, soy, peanuts, green beans, oats, and chocolate. Of course, if you tried to eliminate everything to which you *might* be sensitive, you'd have very little left to eat! Some of my patients who have worked with alternative practitioners have indeed made such radical changes, only to get so bored or frustrated with the same few foods every day that they gave up on their diets entirely.

I think that the best way to find out if you are food-sensitive is to keep a food log, noting what you eat and how you feel within the next thirty to sixty minutes. If you begin to discover that certain foods seem to bring on the feeling of being spacey, tired, or depressed, try one of these strategies:

- *Elimination diet:* Try cutting out the suspected foods entirely for two to four weeks. Then add one back, noting how you feel in your food log. If you are sensitive to the food, you should have a pretty clear reaction, especially if you've gone without it for the suggested time. If you have no negative reaction, you know the food is safe. Repeat this process with each of your suspect foods until you've figured out how your diet affects your mood.

- *Pulse test:* Get a good baseline record of your pulse by checking it several times a day, such as before you get out of bed, before each meal, half an hour after each meal, and before bed. Then, during a testing period of a few days, consume different foods throughout the day, checking your pulse just before you eat and again half an hour later. Record the results. If your pulse increases significantly—by more than eight to ten beats per minute—you may have a food intolerance.

- **Blood test:** You can get a special blood test for food sensitivities pretty easily. These tests are sophisticated and reliable, but they are not cheap. If you're interested, check the resources listed in Appendix C.

Even if you have a food sensitivity, you don't necessarily have to cut the food out of your diet completely. If you avoid your "danger foods" for three to four weeks, your system will probably become less reactive. Then you can reintroduce these "trigger foods" in moderation, not eating any trigger food more than once every four or five days.

5

NATURE'S PHARMACY: SUPPORTING MOOD WITH NUTRITIONAL SUPPLEMENTS AND HERBS

Effective though they may be, diet and exercise are sometimes not enough to overcome depression, especially if you're in the throes of an acute episode. In that case, you might need medication. But if you can manage on nutritional and herbal supplements instead, you'll be duplicating your body's chemistry more closely, with fewer side effects. Dave, Jennifer, and Sarah all benefited from the vitamins, minerals, and other supplements that I describe in this chapter.

You, too, can use supplements to boost your mood and energy levels. I think you need them in three situations:

1. **For Prevention:** You can take vitamins, antioxidants, minerals, and essential fatty acids in lower doses as a general preventive measure. People with high resilience and/or generally good diets may not need to use supplements in this way (though I myself, as a high-resilience person on a good diet, do take them). People with low resilience may be more reliant on them, especially if they have trouble sticking to a healthy diet. *Supplements won't make up for consuming too much sugar, caffeine, and refined carbohydrates, however; nor will they substitute for insufficient healthy carbs.*

2. **During Stressful Times:** When you know you're under stress, you might take vitamins, antioxidants, minerals, and essential fatty acids in moderate doses to help you ward off the likelihood that stress will bring on depression. You can also take 5-HTP, an amino-acid precur-

sor, to help you ward off excess stress. *You should be particularly careful about your diet during these times. Don't expect supplements to compensate for poor diet—they're a boost, not a total remedy.*

3. **During Depressive Episodes:** Here's where you take the highest doses of nutritional supplements, amino-acid precursors, and herbs. *Again, watch your diet most carefully during these times.*

Because I believe you should know what supplements you're taking and why, I've laid out a lot of basic information in this chapter. Note that I haven't given you exact prescriptions, but rather a range of doses. You may need to experiment a little to find out what you need and what feels right. You can either start at the low doses and work your way up or start at the high doses and cut back if you notice any problems or if you feel you're taking too much.

However, if you want to skip right to my recommendations, just look for the boxes below and on pages 81 and 87. They'll tell you basic steps you can take for prevention, during stressful times, or during depressive episodes.

For Prevention: Your Basic Prescription

If you're trying to prevent depression, a good, basic response is to take the key B vitamins in high doses: **10–50 mg daily of B_6, 400 mcg of folic acid, and 20–100 mcg of B_{12} (with up to 500 mcg for the elderly or anyone who absorbs B_{12} poorly).** Your best bet is probably a good B-complex, since a daily multivitamin won't have high enough doses.

You should also add fish-oil supplements to your diet: **an additional 1000 mg** unless you're suffering from acute depression, or if you have an inflammatory-related condition, such as asthma, diabetes, heart disease, arthritis, gum disease, cancer or musculoskeletal injury, and chronic aches and pains, in which case, **increase your dose to 2000 to 3000 mg daily.** If you've been diagnosed with bipolar disorder, **you can take up to 9000 to 10,000 mg per day.** (If you're a vegetarian or just can't bear the thought of fish oil, see the essential fatty acids section below to find out how you can substitute flax-seed oil. Fish oil is better, though, if you can manage it.)

Finally, take the following essential antioxidants, either in a good multivitamin (if you can find one high enough in the recommended doses) or separately:

- *Vitamin C:* 100 to 250 mg twice daily
- *Vitamin E:* 400 mg daily, taken with food
- *Beta-carotene:* taken in a supplement of mixed carotenoids at a daily dose of approximately 25,000 IU
- *Selenium:* 200 mcg daily

NUTRITIONAL SUPPLEMENTS: B VITAMINS, ANTIOXIDANTS, MINERALS, AND ESSENTIAL FATTY ACIDS

Vitamins and minerals are the mildest supplements I recommend in this chapter, and the only ones you can take without consulting with a physician (though I always advise informing your doctor about what you're doing). As we saw in Chapter 4, your brain needs vitamins and minerals to process serotonin, norepinephrine, dopamine, and beta-endorphins, and so to stabilize your mood and energy. Ideally, we'd get all the vitamins and minerals we need from the food we eat, but often we simply don't.

Jennifer, for example, tended to live on a college-student diet of pizza, hamburgers, french fries, and snacks from her dorm's vending machine. No wonder she was lacking in vitamins, minerals, and other essential nutrients! But even Dave, who had spent a lifetime eating healthy home-cooked meals, needed more nutrients to combat his depression than his diet normally included. I prescribed B vitamins and fish-oil supplements to both of them, while advising Jennifer to improve her diet as well.

Eventually, Dave, with his high resilience, could probably dispense with the supplements. Jennifer, with her low resilience, would likely always need to watch her diet carefully and perhaps rely on supplements as well, though in lower, "maintenance" doses as she improved. Both

Dave and Jennifer should resume taking higher doses of supplements when they're under greater stress, however, as well as during times when they're prone to seasonal depression, and at the first signs of a lowering of mood. Women prone to depression should take high doses of supplements while experiencing hormonal changes (PMS, menopause, after childbirth).

B VITAMINS

I think of the Bs as the "antistress vitamin." If you're feeling the strain of an increased workload, a hectic family situation, or a series of setbacks in your personal life, you might consider adding a B-complex to your daily diet, particularly if you drink caffeinated beverages, which, like stress, tend to erode your store of B. While I don't consider myself to have a particularly stressful life, I take a daily B-complex as "stress insurance," a step I often recommend to both high- and low-resilience patients.

Besides their extraordinary assistance with stress and depression, Bs help the brain transform amino acids into such neurotransmitters as serotonin, norepinephrine, and dopamine. And they keep your body from making too much homocysteine, a potentially harmful substance that can promote inflammation. You can simply take a B-complex, or focus on the following B vitamins:

Vitamin B_6: helps in the production of serotonin from the amino acid known as L-tryptophan. Some research suggests that B_6 might help address premenstrual syndrome (PMS), autism, and some seizure disorders, as well as help prevent many chronic diseases associated with inflammation. A study also found that supplementation helped antidepressants work better in an elderly population who also had cognitive dysfunction.[1] **I recommend 10 to 50 mg twice a day of the pyridoxal-5-phosphate (or "pyridoxine"), the active form of B_6.** Ideally, you should take the dosage between meals, but if it causes nausea, take it with food. Be careful not to exceed the recommended dose, particularly because doses over 300 mg daily may lead to peripheral neuropathy (numbness and tingling in the hands and feet).

Folic acid: Studies have shown that 10 to 35 percent of psychiatric patients are low in this crucial vitamin,[2] a deficiency that was even more common among elderly patients. And when patients suffering from depression were given a daily supplement of folic acid, they were better able to function, enjoying better sleep, appetite, mood, motivation, concentration, and energy, and also improving their social functioning, with reduced tendencies to withdraw or isolate themselves and more ability to communicate and sustain important relationships. Another study done by Harvard scientists in 1997 showed that depressed people who had low levels of folic acid were less likely to respond to Prozac than those with normal levels. Folic acid is crucial for the manufacture of neurotransmitters and helps to combat inflammation. **I recommend a dose of 400 mcg daily.**

Vitamin B_{12}: B_{12} and folic acid work together in a powerful combination: Both help the brain produce needed neurotransmitters and help to reduce inflammation. B_{12} can be a powerful antidote to depression: A study published in the *Journal of Psychosomatic Research* found that men who had lost a partner in the last six months suffered more intensely from depression, anxiety, and confusion if their B_{12} levels were low.[3] A study among seven hundred women above the age of sixty-five found a clear correlation between depression and B_{12} deficiency. The more severe the depression, the higher the correlation.[4] And a Finnish study comparing the responses of people with major depression to antidepressants found that people with higher B_{12} levels did relatively better than those with lower levels.[5]

It's particularly important for you to take B_{12} if you're also taking folic acid; otherwise, you risk masking a B_{12} deficiency. **I recommend 20 to 100 mcg daily of B_{12}, with higher doses among the elderly or anyone who absorbs B_{12} poorly—up to 500 mcg daily.** Some people absorb B_{12} more easily when they take it sublingually (under the tongue) or in a nasal spray. People who lack the ability to absorb B_{12} through their gastrointestinal tracts may get B_{12} injections twice weekly for a month and then once or twice a month.

The rest of the Bs are less important for your mood, though they can play a role in combating stress. I suggest either getting a B-complex that contains all of the B vitamins or else looking for a very good multivitamin with adequate doses of B_6, B_{12}, and folic acid.

How to Get the Most from Your Vitamins and Minerals

1. Vitamins are quickly eliminated from the body, so divide your daily dosage into two or more equal parts and take them over the day. In most cases, you can simply take one dose in the morning and another in the evening, or, if you need to take them with meals, with breakfast and dinner.

2. Take all vitamin and mineral supplements with meals if you have any nausea or suffer from any other side effects, as some people do from B vitamins.

3. Tablets may be hard for some people to absorb, so look for "soft-pressed" tablets, liquid, or capsules.

4. Rather than buying all your vitamins and minerals separately, look for a good B-complex along with an antioxidant including vitamin C. Or you can purchase a high-quality multivitamin. Note that in order to get therapeutic doses, you'll need to take two to six pills per day. A once-daily vitamin supplement won't have enough nutrients to treat depression. I recommend any one of the high-quality multivitamin/mineral complexes on the market: Rainbow Light, Twinlab, Natrol, NatureMade, Eclectic Institute, Source Naturals, or the brand put out by Andrew Weil, MD. They can be expensive, but it's still cheaper to buy the complex than to buy each component separately.

ANTIOXIDANTS

Antioxidants are named for their ability to combat *oxidation*, the process by which the by-products of oxygen metabolism may destroy the body's cells, DNA, or other crucial cell structures. Recent evidence suggests that antioxidants help prevent heart disease, cancer, and possibly Alzheimer's disease as well.

Acute depression is one of the most stressful states experienced by human beings. It can be very damaging to brain and other sensitive tissue. So I recommend taking antioxidants to counter the harm from the brain's overexposure to stress hormones.

Some recent research also suggests that depression, like heart disease, is related to an overly sensitive immune-system response and the excessive inflammation that results. A number of inflammatory hormones and other substances are elevated in depression. Antidepressants seem to work as potent anti-inflammatory drugs—but antioxidants, while less intense, have something of the same effect. They, too, help to dampen the inflammatory response, as well as protecting brain tissue. If you're suffering from acute depression, if you're prone to inflammatory diseases (asthma, fibromyalgia, arthritis, Alzheimer's disease, heart disease, diabetes, and gum disease, among others), or if you've got other signs of heightened inflammation (aches and pains from aging or injuries that don't fully heal), you should boost your antioxidant intake right away.

Clearly it is best to get antioxidants from your diet by eating a wide range of fresh fruits and vegetables, particularly those that are bright red, purple, or dark green.[6] But if you're undergoing excessive stress or unable to eat an ideal diet, supplement your daily food intake with the following antioxidants:

- *Vitamin C:* a dose of 100 to 250 mg twice daily
- *Vitamin E:* a dose of 400 mg daily, taken with food
- *Beta-carotene:* taken in a supplement of mixed carotenoids at a daily dose of approximately 15,000 to 25,000 IU
- *Selenium:* 200 mcg daily[7]

MINERALS

In the 1950s, scientists happened upon a discovery that changed the face of psychiatry. They found that lithium, a mineral present in some soils, had a profound effect upon mood, especially agitated states like mania (bipolar disorder). While lithium is the best-known mineral with psychotropic properties, other minerals can also help control depression.

Veterinarians have long observed that aggressive animals became calmer when given a multimineral supplement. Researchers have recently tested that supplement in humans and found that bipolar disorder, both mania and depression, improved significantly. In 2001, psychiatric researcher C.W. Popper described a case of a ten-year-old boy with bipolar disorder and severe tantrums. When the boy began to take the supplement used in farm animals, his symptoms cleared totally. When his family ran out of the supplement a few weeks later, the boy relapsed completely. Then he went on a similar supplement, with partial improvement, and when he got back on the original formula, he again enjoyed a complete remission.

Popper conducted noncontrolled studies with a larger group of twenty-two patients—nineteen of whom improved after taking a multi-mineral supplement. He speculates that there is an interaction between trace mineral and medications that helps the medications work better. Certainly when patients took a mineral supplement, they got by on lower doses of their meds—and enjoyed fewer side effects as a result.[8]

As we saw in Chapter 4, our food supply has become relatively mineral-deficient in recent decades, mostly because of agricultural practices. It could be that Popper's observations are reflecting the effects of subtle mineral deficiencies, which for some people have dramatic effects on mood. Or perhaps there is some sort of genetic metabolic problem that makes some people particularly vulnerable to mood disorders when they don't get enough minerals. Scientists are still trying to figure it out.

Meanwhile, what we do know is that some minerals, including calcium and magnesium, are directly involved in processes whereby neurotransmitters affect our cells. Following is a list of the minerals I think are most important. Most should be present in a good multivitamin/mineral supplement, but you can also just buy these minerals separately:

- *Calcium:* 250 to 500 mg in the morning and 500 to 1000 mg at bedtime
- *Magnesium:* taken with calcium, in a ratio of two parts calcium to one part magnesium
- *Chromium:* 200 to 300 mcg daily
- *Copper and zinc:* taken in a ratio of seven to fifteen parts zinc (up to 30 mg daily) to one part copper (1–2 mg daily)
- *Manganese:* about 5 mg daily

ESSENTIAL FATTY ACIDS

In addition to vitamins and minerals, I'd suggested that Dave take fish-oil capsules to replenish his essential fatty acids (EFAs), which have been shown in many contexts to help patients overcome depression. In places like Japan and Scandinavia, where large amounts of fish are consumed, researchers have found a strong association between fish consumption and lower incidence of depression, suggesting that Omega-3 EFAs have a protective effect.[9] And as we saw in Chapter 4, our dietary changes over the past hundred years have dramatically transformed the ratio of Omega-3 to Omega-6 fatty acids from about 1:1 in our ancestors to our current ratio of 1:25, putting us at a vastly higher risk of inflammation and its related diseases, possibly including depression.[10] Indeed, as we saw in Chapter 1, rates of depression have risen steadily over the past century. So even though we don't yet know exactly how EFAs affect brain chemistry, clearly they do.

Thus, at a recent symposium sponsored by the National Institutes of Mental Health (NIMH) devoted entirely to the therapeutic use of fats in mental illness, several presenters reported the beneficial effects of EFA supplementation on depression, bipolar illness, and schizophrenia. Adding EFAs to the diets of research subjects has been associated with improvements in dyslexia and attention deficit hyperactivity disorder (ADHD) as well as improved intelligence measures in ten-month-olds and in adults with Alzheimer's disease.[11]

More significantly for our purposes, EFAs were also reported to reduce anxiety levels in students preparing for exams,[12] while studies on schizophrenics found that patients treated with EFA supplements showed a reduction even in their severe symptoms: delusions, aggressive hostility, and mood swings—as well as improvements in memory and cognitive function.[13] In a similar 1999 study reported in the *Archives of General Psychiatry*[14] high doses of fish oil were given to bipolar patients in addition to their usual medications. After four months, three times as many patients on the EFA supplements had lower levels of depression and other psychiatric symptoms than those who had been given placebos. Finally, researchers in England found that red-blood-cell levels of DHA and EPA—two essential fatty acids—were lower in depressed and schizophrenic patients than in mentally healthy research subjects—further evidence that there is a link between these dietary fats and mental health.[15]

Why would relatively small amounts of these healthy fats have an effect on mood? One possibility is that there is some kind of connection between excessive or chronic inflammation and depression. It has been shown that certain inflammatory substances, eicosanoids and cytokines, are elevated in major depression. These elements promote low-level inflammation, which may affect brain tissue as well as other parts of the body. Antidepressants suppress this harmful activity, but so can increased levels of Omega-3s, and probably more efficiently.[16]

Finally, in addition to their role in inflammatory processes, the Omega-3 fatty acids are also important for proper nerve cell function. As we saw in Chapter 4, these fats become part of the nerve cell membrane and are important for keeping the cell and their receptors working efficiently. Since receptors are the "lock" into which the neurotransmitter "key" fits, anything that supports receptor function will help the brain better distribute neurochemicals to promote mood.

There is also evidence that fatty acids have a more direct effect on neurotransmitters. People who get more Omega-3s seem to have higher levels of serotonin and dopamine by-products in their spinal fluid, suggesting that their brain levels of these vital neurochemicals are also higher.[17]

Indeed, Dave responded well to fish-oil supplements. Like most Americans, he rarely ate healthy fat and was probably among the norm who have an Omega-3–Omega-6 ratio of about 1:25. While this didn't cause his depression, it may have left him more vulnerable than usual to the stresses that he experienced. Boosting his Omega-3 levels definitely created a healthier environment in his brain and central nervous system, "preparing the soil" so that the other measures we took could work.

Fish oil: Toxins and heavy metals may become concentrated in fish fat, so look for "molecular distilled" products. Fish oils are best if you also eat foods high in EFAs, such as fish, flax, pumpkin seeds, and nuts—particularly walnuts, but also almonds, macadamia nuts, Brazil nuts, cashews, and pistachios. Follow the dietary recommendations I suggested in Chapter 4, and then supplement your diet with **an additional 1000 mg of Omega-3.** (Add together the amounts of DHA and EPA listed on the supplement you buy to make sure you're getting 1000 mg, which is typically three to four capsules daily.) If you're suffering from acute depression, or if you have an inflammatory-related condition, such as asthma, diabetes, heart disease, arthritis, gum disease, cancer or musculoskeletal injury, and chronic aches and pains, you can **increase your dose to 2000 to 3000 mg daily.** If you've been diagnosed with bipolar disorder, **the recommended dose is 7500 to 10,000 mg per day.** If you really can't bear the thought of eating fish or fish oil, read on to see my recommendations for flax seed.

Flaxseed: This is another source of Omega-3 fatty acids, and it can be a good addition to your diet, or a substitute for fish and fish oil. Although flaxseed doesn't contain the essential Omega-3 DHA and EPA, as fish oil does, your body can theoretically convert the elements of flaxseed oil into these other EFAs. However, some people's bodies have trouble making this conversion, rendering flaxseed oil slightly less effective than fish/fish oil for some people, so I still recommend fish oil over flaxseed oil if possible.

If you are using flaxseed oil, **take one to two capsules twice a day or one tablespoon of flax oil each day.** I recommend Barlean's Flax Oil or Health from the Sun "Total EFA," which has a mixture of oils, not just flax. If you're taking oil rather than capsules, keep the liquid refrigerated, and—since some manufacturing methods can destroy the nutrient value—make sure you buy only opaque bottles of oil marked "expeller-pressed at low temperatures." The methods I prefer go by proprietary names such as Bio-Electron Process, Spectra-Vac, and Omegaflo.

Ground flaxseeds: are an alternative to flaxseed oil. You can grind them in a coffee grinder and then store them in the refrigerator in an airtight container. I personally prefer ground flaxseeds to any of the oils: They're cheaper, they taste better, and the seed form enables you to get the fiber and healthy lignans from the seeds. Mix them into juice or a smoothie, or sprinkle them over cereal or a salad. Eat about two tablespoons per day.

Evening primrose, borage seed, or black currant oils: These are good sources of gamma-linoleic acid (GLA), which improves the effectiveness of both fish and flaxseed oils. I recommend taking these in addition to fish oil if you have signs of inflammation or if you have a diet high in Omega-6 fatty acids (which most Americans do, especially if they eat nonorganic beef, chicken, and eggs; organic grass- or flax-fed animal products are higher in Omega-3s). **Doses range up to 2800 mg in arthritis studies. If you are also taking fish or flax oil, you should be able to take between 150 and 500 mg of GLA daily with good results.**

During Stressful Times: Your Basic Prescription

If you're under a lot of stress, having particular problems with sleep, or fit the description of serotonin deficiency in the chart below, you might go for a more intense supplement along with your vitamins or minerals. Try 5-HTP, a precursor to tryptophan, the amino acid that your brain uses to produce serotonin. Start slowly: **only 50 mg at night.** If you don't notice any side effects after a few days, **up your dose to 150 mg at night if helpful for sleep, or else just take 50 to 100 mg three times a day.**

Warning: *Do NOT take 5-HTP if you are also taking a prescription antidepressant. Do NOT stop taking a prescription medication in order to take 5-HTP. Inform the physician who is treating your depression and/or prescribing medication before beginning to take 5-HTP.*

Which Amino Acids Do You Need?

Signs of serotonin deficiency suggesting a need to supplement with 5-HTP:
- depressed or irritable mood
- insomnia and anxiety
- binge eating or carbohydrate craving
- restless energy and an overactive mind
- feelings of insecurity or impulsivity
- low tolerance or overreactivity to stress

Signs of norepinephrine deficiency suggesting a need to supplement with DL-phenylalanine:
- depressed mood
- increased sleep
- fatigue, sluggishness, or lethargy
- poor attention or memory
- apathy

Signs of dopamine deficiency suggesting a need to supplement with L-tyrosine:

- depressed mood
- excessive sleeping
- weight gain or obesity
- lack of energy
- lack of enjoyment or pleasure
- low sexual interest
- nicotine addiction

Warning: Do NOT *take amino-acid supplements without informing your physician.* **Do NOT** *take amino-acid supplements if you are already taking prescription antidepressants. Remember that amino-acid supplements can be potent, especially at higher doses, and can interact with other substances, especially prescription antidepressants.*

⟆⟋⟍⟍⟍⟍⟍⟍⟍9

AMINO-ACID PRECURSORS

Sarah, whom we met in Chapter 3, was especially sensitive to stress and seemed to have a poorly functioning serotonin system. I imagined her "serotonin tank" being rather small and only half-full most of the time. That could be improved with many of the preventive measures in this book, but I knew that she would likely go through periods in her life when unforeseen stress got the better of her and her serotonin level would dip below that imaginary line where symptoms of depression appear.

As we saw, Sarah didn't want to go on medication, a choice with which I agreed. I thought she could stay off meds if she agreed to respond quickly to her biochemical imbalance, taking immediate measures to boost her serotonin supply to healthy levels. I felt confident that she could achieve that goal with amino-acid precursors, particularly if she hadn't become severely depressed.

Amino acids are the basic constituents of protein, and they're what the brain uses to make neurotransmitters. Because proteins contain so many amino acids, these crucial elements often "compete" with one another in their efforts to be absorbed by the brain. As a result, the amino acids that are most important for regulating mood often don't make it into the brain in sufficiently high levels. Tryptophan, the building block for serotonin, has a particularly difficult time reaching the appropriate parts of the brain. As they did for Sarah, amino-acid supplements can thus help many patients manufacture the brain chemicals they need to overcome depression.

Maximizing Benefits from Amino Acids

If you're taking any of the amino-acid supplements described below, you'll want to take them at least thirty minutes before you eat, since you'll absorb amino acids better without competition from any other protein. Capsules are better absorbed than tablets.

Amino acids work almost like medication, so I advise you to use them as cautiously as you would any prescription drug, ideally under the supervision of a trained practitioner. If you're already taking antidepressants or any other type of medication, don't take any amino acid without an expert's recommendation and supervision, since the combinations can present some risk.

5-HYDROXYTRYPTOPHAN (5-HTP)

Extracted from an African plant called *Griffonia simplificolia*, 5-HTP is converted into serotonin in the brain. When you eat trytophan-bearing foods, your brain converts the amino acid into 5-HTP, and from that, makes serotonin. Taking a 5-HTP supplement is thus another way to boost your serotonin levels.

5-HTP dissolves more easily in the body's fat cells than tryptophan does, so it gets into the brain more easily. Taking 5-HTP may have an even more beneficial effect than antidepressants because instead of merely preventing the recycling of serotonin, 5-HTP actually increases serotonin levels. Several studies from the 1970s and 1980s found that about two-thirds of the patients studied had good responses to 5-HTP.[18] And among people who did not respond well to antidepressants, the response rate was still as high as 50 percent, which compared favorably to other medical treatments.[19] A more recent Swiss study, comparing 5-HTP to Luvox, a newer antidepressant, found that the patients taking 5-HTP had a greater decrease in depression, anxiety, somatic pain, and insomnia than the Luvox group, with better rates of tolerance for the supplement than for the medication.[20] 5-HTP has also been studied over a two-year period in depressed patients, revealing that the supplement is effective in helping to prevent relapse into depression.[21]

Some mild side effects can result from 5-HTP—further bearing out its similarity to medications. Most common side effects include nausea, cramping, and diarrhea. Some patients, whose serotonin receptors have become more sensitive than normal in order to make the best possible use of low serotonin levels, experience a degree of anxiety when they start taking 5-HTP, as the body is overly sensitive to the new, higher levels of serotonin. (See the discussion of "up-regulation" in Chapter 3.) Usually, within a couple of weeks, the serotonin receptors become a bit less sensitive and the patient experiences a new sense of well-being and calm.

Unlike the SSRIs, 5-HTP is not associated with sexual side effects or weight gain. In fact, the supplement may actually improve sexual function while reducing food cravings and binge eating.

Until a few years ago, 5-HTP was available only by prescription and was very expensive, making it difficult for most people to use. Now you can get 5-HTP in health-food stores. A moderate dose—150 mg daily—costs only about thirty dollars per month.

I suggest starting slow on this potent supplement: **50 mg at night, increasing to 150 mg at night if helpful for sleep, or 50 to 100 mg three times a day.** If you are having trouble sleeping, take most of this supplement at night (up to 150 mg), unless you find it somehow worsens your sleep (as with antidepressants, amino-acid supplements often have paradoxical or contradictory effects, resulting from the difficulty in *balancing* brain chemistry rather than simply boosting biochemical levels). If you're taking more than 150 mg daily, consume the rest of your 5-HTP during the day. If sleep isn't a problem for you, just divide your 5-HTP doses equally throughout the day. If you're concerned about excessive appetite or binge eating, and if you can tolerate the supplement without nausea, take it about half an hour before meals to help reduce appetite and binge eating. If you find that 5-HTP causes nausea, it may be taken with food. Taking B vitamins with 5-HTP, especially B_6

and folic acid, as well as taking magnesium, may help 5-HTP work more efficiently, as these vitamins and minerals are essential cofactors in the conversion of 5-HTP to serotonin.

DL-PHENYLALANINE AND L-TYROSINE

Phenylalanine is converted into tyrosine, the parent compound for adrenaline, norepinephrine, and phenylethylamine (PEA). PEA is an amphetamine-like compound found in chocolate, which may partially explain the common craving for chocolate as an antidote to depression. This supplement might also help people addicted to stimulation overcome their emotional cravings, and it might work as an alternative to such stimulants as Ritalin in ADHD. It can also be helpful in overcoming pain and inflammation and in achieving withdrawal from stimulating drugs.

The precursor for norepinephrine comes in two forms: D-phenylalanine and L-phenylalanine. Most stores carry just the L-form, but the D-form is more easily converted in the brain. It is more expensive, but you don't need to take as much. I usually recommend buying DL-phenylalanine, a combination of the two, if it can be found. Studies have shown that it compares favorably to antidepressants in its effectiveness.[22]

Some people prefer to take L-tyrosine to directly increase dopamine levels, but there is less evidence that this strategy works for depression. Since the brain can convert phenylalanine into tyrosine, and then tyrosine into dopamine, it may be that the same supplement could enhance both neurotransmitters. The supplement is reportedly helpful in coping with PMS and overcoming chronic fatigue.[23]

I recommend starting with 500 mg daily, early in the day, taken about half an hour before breakfast and lunch. **The dose can be gradually increased, every three to four days (up to 2000–3000 mg daily),** until a response becomes apparent or side effects appear. Some studies have found good effects resulting from much higher doses, but I don't recommend the increase as you run the risk of increased blood pressure and heart rate. Even in moderate doses, you may experience such side effects as overstimulation, anxiety, insomnia, hypertension, stomach upset, and headaches, but these are usually mild and go away if you wait a few days. Taking this supplement with food also helps to reduce its side effects. But if the side effects are unpleasant, or if they persist after three or four days, I usually recommend that my patients back down on the dose and stop altogether if there has been no real benefit.

Be sure to take the dosages of B vitamins and C recommended above along with this supplement, as the vitamins will increase the amino acid's effectiveness.

"SAMe" (S-ADENOSYL-L-METHIONINE)

Naturally occurring throughout the body, SAMe is produced by the brain from the amino acid methionine. SAMe helps increase brain levels of serotonin and dopamine, and it may also improve their ability to attach to their receptors. Although the supplement has only recently become available in the United States, SAMe has been heavily studied and used in Europe since 1975. Some research recommends it to help patients overcome lethargy, apathy, guilt and suicidal feelings, or to overcome strongly obsessive and suicidal tendencies. The supplement is also said to relieve arthritis, fibromyalgia, liver disease, and even Alzheimer's, and it may be more effective in severe depression than St. John's wort.[24]

A 1988 study published in the *American Journal of Psychiatry* focusing on sixty-seven patients with severe depression reported a 50 percent reduction of symptoms in two weeks when patients were given 400 mg of this supplement per day.[25] Other research has shown that the supplement works more rapidly than the antidepressant imipramine, and a large analysis of the research concluded that it is at least as effective as the tricyclic antidepressants. Many of those studies used high doses of SAMe, but it may also work at lower doses.[26]

I recommend a starting dose of 200 mg twice daily, preferably taken thirty minutes before meals or two hours after eating. It may be slowly increased up to 800 mg twice a day if tolerated. A response is usually evident in four to fifteen days. SAMe appears to be quite safe even in long-term use, though it can cause mild headaches, nausea, and excessive stimulation, and it's **definitely not for use by bipolar patients;** it can elevate their mood and cause mania.

It's best to take SAMe with vitamins B_6, B_{12}, folic acid, magnesium, and calcium. These help it work better and reduce any side-effect risks. Because this supplement is highly unstable, buy it in the form of enteric-coated tablets stored in foil packets and keep the pills in the foil until just before you take them.

Another option is to take SAMe with antidepressants, whose effectiveness it may enhance, making them work faster and possibly at lower doses. However, there is a risk that interaction between SAMe and some drugs may have dangerous side effects, so it should be used with caution and only under medical supervision.

Unfortunately, SAMe is quite expensive. When taken in doses high enough to treat more severe depression, it can cost as much as $160 to $320 per month. But doses of 400–800 mg daily are helpful for many patients, at a cost of $40 to $80 per month.

During Depressive Episodes: Your Basic Prescription

For mild depression:

If you have a mild depression, especially with anxiety, you could begin with a trial of St. John's wort. **Take 300 mg of St. John's wort three times daily.** Make sure it is standardized to 0.3 percent hypericin or 5 percent hyperforin, and it should be a "guaranteed potency herb."

If you see little improvement in four weeks, you may increase the dose to 1200 mg daily.

You should also be taking the nutritional supplements in the box on page 71 entitled "For Prevention: Your Basic Prescription."

You can combine St. John's wort with a low dose of the appropriate amino acid. Look at the chart entitled "Which Amino Acid Should You Take?" on page 81 to find out which amino acid is right for you.

Give this combination four to eight weeks to work. If you see no benefit, or if your depression is getting worse, consult your doctor.

For mild to moderate depression:

If you have mild to moderate depression, especially with sluggishness or lethargy, you may want to try SAMe. Begin with **200 mg taken at least a half hour before breakfast, and if you tolerate it well, increase to 400 mg after four days.** Make sure it comes in individual foil packets to preserve freshness.

If there is little improvement in two weeks, you may increase the dose to 800 mg daily.

You should also be taking the nutritional supplements in the shaded box on page 71 entitled "For Prevention: Your Basic Prescription."

You can combine SAMe with a low dose of the appropriate amino acid. Look at the chart entitled "Which Amino Acid Should You Take?" on page 81 to find out which amino acid is right for you.

Give this combination two to four weeks to work. If you see no benefit, or if your depression is getting worse, consult your doctor.

For severe depression, consult your physician. Do NOT try to rely on self-medication during severe depression.

HERBAL THERAPIES

Warning: While herbs are generally considered safe and have fewer reported side effects than medications, you should approach them with the same caution you'd employ in dealing with prescription drugs. After all, if they're strong enough to have potent effects on your body, brain, and mood, they're powerful enough to be treated with respect. Remember, too, that most street drugs are "natural" plant-based products. "Natural" in no way means "safe." I recommend working with a qualified herbalist or other health professional trained in their use.

Herbal medicines have a long tradition around the world, and many herbs have been traditionally used for various kinds of depression or anxiety. Some of these traditional medicines have come into use among alternative and complementary physicians, and even among some conventional doctors.

I personally believe that some herbs have properties similar to prescription medications: They can be effective but must be used with caution. In general, I think that they are milder, with fewer side effects and risks than medication, but there are exceptions. For instance, kava kava was recently taken off the market because of an association with liver failure. St. John's wort has a few notable interactions with other medications. The trend in medicine is to look for a single chemical action to have the desired effect. But in herbal therapies, there can be dozens, if not hundreds, of active constituents in a single plant. This makes herbs more complex, but may also explain some of their effectiveness, because of the way the chemicals work synergistically. Centuries of use should allay some of the fears about herbs, and researchers are now looking at them diligently. In my experience, they can be useful adjuncts in moderately severe depression, and I know that many people respond well to herbs alone for milder depression.

The most notable herb currently in use to treat depression and anxiety is St. John's wort, though some others—including gingko biloba and valerian root—may also be effective in some cases.

St. John's wort (*Hypericum perforatum*): This herb is frequently used in Europe, particularly Germany, where it is prescribed twenty times more often than Prozac. Research suggests that St. John's wort is more effective than placebo and as effective as some medications, with fewer side effects.[27]

However, many physicians and scientists believe that the European research was not rigorous by U.S. scientific standards. Critics also point out that many of the results were subjective—based on patients' judgments rather than observable fact—and that the trials lasted only four to six weeks, not long enough to really treat depression. Moreover, the antidepressants that were being compared to St. John's wort were administered in low doses, and the patients in the studies were diagnosed by primary-care doctors rather than by psychiatrists, who would have been more likely to observe subtleties in symptoms. When more stringent criteria are used, the critics say, St. John's wort appears only 1.5 times more likely to produce a positive response than a placebo.[28]

Most of the research on St. John's wort concerned mild depression, so we didn't really know how it affected more serious instances of depression or anxiety—until recently. The National Institutes of Health (NIH) conducted a major trial, comparing St. John's wort with Zoloft and placebo in the treatment of severe depression, and the results were disappointing. Many supporters of herbal medicine have questioned the study's methods and findings, but it does call into question the effectiveness of St. John's wort as a treatment for depression.[29]

Personally, I don't believe this herb is effective for severe depression by itself, but it may be useful for mild to moderate depression, especially with anxiety. It also may become more effective when used in combination with other treatments.

St. John's wort is well tolerated by most people and considered safe, but it may cause photosensitivity—sensitivity to light, including easy sunburning, as well as headaches, nausea, fatigue, light-headedness, and dry mouth. **Never mix St. John's wort with alcohol or with antidepressants;** its most serious side effect might result from a combination of St. John's wort and SSRIs, which might cause "serotonin syndrome," an excess of serotonin function leading to an altered mental state, twitching or tremors, sweating, flushing, ataxia (unsteadiness on your feet), gastrointestinal upset, headache, myalgia, and restlessness. This can be a serious condition that should receive immediate medical attention. Concerns have also been raised recently by reports that St. John's wort caused other medications to work less effectively—including birth-control pills! Finally, **St. John's wort may induce mania in bipolar patients.**

Most St. John's wort products have been standardized to contain 0.3 percent hypericin, which was once thought to be the active component. You may also see it standardized to 5 percent hyperforin, which is more recently thought to be the therapeutic ingredient. Look for a brand that offers "guaranteed potency."

For mild to moderate depression, I recommend 900–1200 mg daily, spread out over two or three doses. I don't recommend using this herb as the sole treatment for severe depression. Plan on a lag time of about three to four weeks before you begin to feel any effects. It may take even longer.

Ginkgo biloba: This herb does not seem to offer any benefits to healthy adults, but it may be helpful to people with various disorders, including dementia and depression, and seems to be somewhat effective in treating the sexual dysfunction that often appears as a side effect of antidepressants. Some doctors prescribe it along with an SSRI. It seems to work by enhancing microcirculation, improving blood flow to the tiny capillaries to the brain and elsewhere.

Hundreds of studies have been published on ginkgo biloba. In the most rigorous studies, seven out of eight people showed significant improvements in concentration, memory, and depression.[30] A major study in the *Journal of the American Medical Association* published in 1997 found that ginkgo helped patients stabilize and improve their functioning over a period of six months to a year.[31] A 2000 study found the herb had some ability to delay the progression of Alzheimer's disease.[32] And the *Journal of Sex and Marital Therapy* reported in 1998 that ginkgo had a 91 percent success rate in women and 76 percent in men who had experienced SSRI-induced sexual side effects, though in my own practice, I haven't seen results that were nearly that good.[33]

Few side effects have been reported for ginkgo biloba, except for some headaches and mild nausea. However, you should know that this herb may keep blood platelets from clotting, which prolongs bleeding time in case of injury, resulting in two reported cases of ginkgo-related hemorrhage. Definitely avoid taking ginkgo biloba if you have bleeding problems, are taking anticoagulants (Coumadin, vitamin E, and aspirin, among others), or are planning any medical procedures.

I think ginkgo can be a helpful adjunct in the treatment of depression, especially for the depressed elderly, or for someone with significant cognitive symptoms, such as poor memory or concentration. **I recommend a dose of 40 to 60 mg (standardized to 24 percent ginkgo flavone glycosides) three times daily (with food). Or to simplify, you can take 60 to 80 mg of ginkgo biloba twice daily.** I recommend Ginkgold (Nature's Way) and Ginkoba (Pharmaton), the brands used in the European studies. Be prepared for the herb to take several weeks to work.

6

FLOWING WITH NATURE: MOVEMENT, BREATHING, AND BIORHYTHMS

Even though I live among many farmers and people who work on the land, I'm struck by how far all of us have moved from the earth's natural rhythms and cycles. Just a few generations ago, most people lived much closer to the earth. Their daily lives brought them plenty of exercise as a matter of course. Without gaslight or electricity, they slept while it was dark and so they got plenty of rest. Farmers and other rural people lived in harmony with the rhythms of nature, working longer hours in the summer and "hibernating" in the cold, punishing winter. Even many people in cities had jobs requiring hard manual labor, while all but the very rich tended to adjust their lifestyles to the natural world, eating only foods that were in season, for example, and going to bed earlier in winter and later in summer.

But our developing technology has changed all that. Although in many ways, this technology has freed us, we're now living out of sync with the natural rhythms that our animal bodies continue to crave. I believe that ignoring these natural cycles is one of the most significant forces behind today's epidemic of mood and anxiety disorders. Understanding our relationship to *exercise, breathing, biorhythms, sleep,* and *the seasons* can make the difference between a balanced, calm, and happy life, or an existence burdened with stress, anxiety, and depression.

MOVEMENT AS THERAPY

Remember Mary, whom we met in Chapter 4? Although changes in her diet combined with supplements had enabled her to cut her daily dose of Paxil in half, she still felt stuck. Exercise, I told Mary, would put her body in touch with the rhythms of the natural world.

Mary had slipped into another type of vicious cycle. The less active she was, the more weight she gained, and the weaker and less flexible she became. Her posture, too, became more and more slumped, throwing her back and hips out of alignment. The further she declined, the harder she found it to exercise—and the more her risk of injury increased. Less exercise intensified her depression—which only made her feel more sluggish and less interested in moving. Mary tried again to exercise, but again she found herself with a slight injury almost as soon as she'd started running. Ironically, her sore hips proved to be a blessing in disguise, for they led her to a wonderful physical therapist specializing in women's health issues who gave Mary some stretches and strengthening exercises to help stabilize her trunk—her hips, back, abdomen, chest, and neck.

Gradually, Mary gained strength and her posture improved. She also found that she could move without pain, until she was eventually able to do a combination walk/jog of one and a half to two miles a few times a week. Stretches and strength-training exercises were also a key part of her routine.

Three months later when Mary came to see me, she was positively beaming. "Well, doctor, I've got a bone to pick with you," she said, barely able to keep the grin from breaking through. "I've lost so much weight that I've got to go out and buy all new clothes. It's going to cost me a fortune to get a smaller wardrobe!" Mary felt lighter—physically, mentally, and spiritually—than she'd felt in thirty years.

Exercise: The Wonder Drug

Exercise has so many benefits in combating depression and improving brain chemistry that the following advice—while true—may sound like a cliché: Find a form of vigorous movement that appeals to you, practice it three to five times a week for twenty to forty minutes, and watch your mood improve. In fact, there's so much powerful research on the health and mood benefits of exercise that I sometimes wonder why they keep funding more studies! If a new drug came on the market that helped depression as much as exercise does, you can believe that patients would be clamoring for their doctors to prescribe it. Yet exercise is free, available to all, and (if you do it right) has no unpleasant side effects, only beneficial ones. If you take away only one message from this book, let it be this one: **Getting regular, vigorous exercise is the best possible way that you can alter your own brain chemistry and improve your mood.**

I could fill this entire book with a summary of the research showing the benefits of exercise. Here are only a few of the most dramatic results:

- In 1978, Dr. John Greist did a study showing that running was as effective as psychotherapy in treating depression.[1]

- In 1984, researchers I. L. McCann and D. S. Holmes studied three groups of depressed women, one of which did aerobic exercise, another of which did relaxing exercise, and the last of which did no exercise. Only the first, the aerobic group, showed a steady decrease in depression.[2]

- A 1999 study by researchers at Duke University who later published their results in the *Archives of Internal Medicine* compared exercise, medication, and a combination of the two among a group of 156 middle-aged and elderly patients with nonsuicidal depression. The medication involved was Zoloft, a very effective means of treating depression, while the exercise program consisted of a thrice-weekly forty-five-minute class that included thirty minutes of brisk walking or jogging. To the researchers' amazement, after sixteen weeks, all three groups showed similar improvements.[3]

- A follow-up to this study, published in *Psychosomatic Medicine* in 2000[4] checked back on how the patients were doing six months after the initial study. The exercise-only group was actually doing better than the other two: Fewer than one-third of the med-free exercisers had relapsed back into depression, compared to over half of the patients in the meds and meds/exercise groups.

Why does exercise affect your brain chemistry so much? Well, to be honest, we're not exactly sure. But here are some of the possible reasons:

- Increased body temperature leads to a more relaxed state.
- Deeper breathing and increased heart rate lead to greater blood flow and oxygenation of the brain and other vital organs, which in turn provide more energy and nutrients to the cells and clear more toxins from your system.

- Exercise increases your brain's ability to create and utilize the vital chemicals serotonin, dopamine, and norepinephrine.
- The release of certain brain chemicals, including endorphins and another category known as enkephalins, leads to a greater sense of well-being.
- Exercise increases the availability of such stress hormones as cortisol, boosting our ability to respond to stress.

Exercise is one of those treatments we physicians love, especially when we're dealing with depression, because it has both physical and emotional benefits. In other words, your health improves—and you feel better, too.

Emotional Benefits of Exercise

- helps alleviate stress and anxiety
- increases self-confidence and a sense of mastery and control
- distracts from negative thoughts and feelings—it's hard to feel depressed while exercising
- elevates mood
- boosts serotonin levels over a prolonged period of time
- improves stress tolerance—it's like getting a stress immunization
- may involve positive social interactions; mitigates against isolation and withdrawal

In combination with antidepressants, exercise
- improves blood circulation to the brain, helping the medication get to where it is needed
- may improve metabolism, allowing for a lower dosage of medication
- reduces the sexual side effects of medication
- helps control medication-related weight gain and fatigue

In many cases, regular aerobic exercise, sometimes supplemented by strength training, enables depressed patients either to avoid medication or to get off it entirely. Even if, like Mary, it's best for you to continue your antidepressant medication, exercise can help your meds work better and reduce their side effects.

Warning: If you have any physical limitations, or if it has been a long time since you have exercised, consult your doctor before beginning any exercise program. But do begin! No matter how old you are or what your physical status, there is some kind of exercise you can do with the right kind of guidance and supervision. Even wheelchair-bound amputees can exercise—and so can you. In fact, exercise is all the more crucial if you are older or disabled in any way, both to support your physical health and to boost your mood.

Your Brain-Healthy Exercise Plan: Exercising for Improved Mental Health

- Find an aerobic exercise that you enjoy and engage in it for thirty minutes every day—or sixty minutes if you are trying to lose weight. Note that we're talking about thirty or sixty minutes *total*, so you might, for example, walk part of the way to work (ten minutes), take a brisk lunchtime walk (ten minutes), and then walk part of the way home (ten minutes). Note that even a ten-minute period of activity has been proven to lift mood, so even if you have time only for a short walk, try to do *something*.[5]
- If you can, add strength training, especially if you suffer from "sluggish depression" (shortages of norepinephrine/dopamine), tend to be overweight, or are an Earth/kapha type (see Chapters 7 and 10).
- Note that aerobic exercise seems to be better at reducing anxiety, while weight training helps boost self-esteem. So try to engage in some of each, adjusting the balance to your own personal needs.
- If you're suffering from a low-serotonin depression, do serotonin-boosting activities, such as yoga, stretching, tai chi, qigong, and other types of gentle exercise. Generally, you might follow the recommendations for the Air/vata type (see Chapters 7 and 8).
- If you're suffering from an agitated depression—excess dopamine combined with low serotonin levels, you'll benefit from the calming effects of tai chi, the cooling effects of swimming, and the vigorous, stress-busting effects of brisk walking, skiing, skating, rowing, canoeing, tennis, and golf, though you should avoid situations in which your exercise

is competitive rather than simply energetic. Follow the recommendations for the Fire/pitta type (see Chapters 7 and 9).

- If your problem is a shortage of dopa/norepi, engage in more vigorous, stimulating exercise, such as aerobics classes, running, and weight training. Follow the recommendations for the Earth/kapha type (see Chapters 7 and 10).

- If, like Mary, your posture is stooped over or your chest is closed, explore yoga stretches that open the heart chakra, such as backward bends and chest openers (cobra, locust, camel, backbend).

- Keep exercising even after your depression is improved. As the Duke University study showed, maintaining a regular exercise schedule may make the difference in whether or not you have a relapse. Although you may someday be able to stop taking antidepressants, exercise—and proper diet—are a lifelong commitment, especially if you are prone to depression. So start finding ways to integrate vigorous movement into your life. It really is the best medicine for body, mind, and spirit.

THE BREATH OF LIFE

Breathing is integral to our lives, and conscious breathing—breathing done with awareness—can be a terrific way of altering our mood, overcoming depression, anxiety, and sleeplessness. Proper breathing helps to integrate our body, mind, and spirit. It's also crucial to our brain chemistry. Think of what happens when you get angry. Your breath comes forcefully, aggressively pushing your words and feelings out into the world. When you're scared, on the other hand, your breath tends to be shallow and restricted, while we can read one another's sadness in the spasmodic inward breathing of a sigh or a sob.

Because your breath and your mental/emotional state are so closely linked, changing one will change the other. In other words, calming yourself after an angry shouting match or a sorrowful burst of tears will result in slower, more even breathing. But slowing your breathing will also help to calm you down.

The key to all breathing practice is *abdominal breathing*, in which the breath is drawn deep into the abdomen, which moves freely. I recommend practicing this vital technique for five to ten minutes a day, until it becomes automatic. Then you can draw on the Calming Breath Technique and the Energizing Breath Technique as needed.

Abdominal Breath Technique

- Sit comfortably, with your back upright but not rigid and your eyes open; or, lie on your back, with your knees up or supported by a pillow.
- Place a hand on your lower abdomen.
- Put the tip of your tongue on your palate, just behind and above your teeth.
- Breathe through your nose. This takes a little practice (and you may not be able to do it if you're congested), but nose breathing is a terrific way to channel oxygen right into the brain, with marvelous effects on your brain chemistry.
- Focus your attention on your belly, just below your navel.
- Relax and soften the muscles of your abdomen.
- Feel the breath float in, pushing your belly out. Visualize drawing your breath all the way down into your lower abdomen.
- Feel your breath float out, pulling your belly in. Again, exhale from your lower abdomen.
- Allow your chest and shoulders to relax so that you have more movement in your abdomen than in your upper body.
- Sit or lie still for a few minutes, keeping your belly soft, noticing how your abdomen rises and falls as you breathe.
- Try to deepen and slow your breath, breathing in on a count of eight or twelve, and breathing out on the same count.

WHEN YOU FEEL ANXIOUS . . .

You can use the following Calming Breath Technique whenever you get anxious or if you have difficulty sleeping. I also recommend practicing it for ten minutes each day no matter what, especially if you think your depression is related to low serotonin levels.

⌘

Calming Breath Technique

- Slowly breathe in through your nose.
- Hold your breath for a few seconds.
- Breathe out even more slowly through your mouth. Try to make your exhalation take longer than your inhalation. You may structure your breathing, if you'd like, by counting to four as you breathe in, to two as you hold the breath, and to seven as you breathe out. Some people find it even more calming to make an audible sigh with their outbreath.

⌘

WHEN YOU FEEL SLUGGISH . . .

You can also use your breath to increase your energy and mental clarity. Breathing vigorously, as you do when you exercise, raises heart rate, increases blood flow, and aids in the release of hormones, signaling to your body and mind that they need to rise to the challenge, becoming more alert and ready for action. Use the Energizing Breath Technique whenever your energy sags, your mind dulls, or you don't feel fully awake. And if you've got the sluggish type of depression that may come from a dopamine/norepinephrine deficiency, I recommend practicing this technique for about a minute several times a day.

⌘

Energizing Breath Technique

- Breathe in and out as fast as you can.
- Make your inbreath and outbreath of equal lengths.
- Do this for fifteen to twenty seconds at first, progressing up to a minute or more with practice.
- Reduce the duration of the practice if light-headedness occurs.

⌘

ACTIVITY AND REST:
THE BODY'S NEED FOR BALANCE

Surely we humans are the only creatures who refuse to rest after periods of intense or prolonged activity. Our bodies crave the natural rhythm of vigorous activity followed by rest and relaxation—but how many of us work long hours with no breaks, even using our lunch hours, evenings, and weekends to catch up on paperwork, make cell-phone calls, or do the million and one errands that have piled up during the week? No wonder the incidence of depression is on the rise!

After two decades of practicing psychiatry, I have come to believe that this unremitting busy-ness is one of the major causes of a general breakdown of resilience. I had a dramatic illustration of the need for rest and renewal early in my career, when I had what I thought was the golden opportunity of working as medical director of the mental-health department for a very large HMO. I was responsible for more than one hundred professional staff who served more than 300,000 HMO members. It was a huge and complex job, but I found it interesting and challenging and very much wanted to do it.

At the same time, though, I was practicing psychiatry nearly full-time, I was married, and I was committed to being an active parent to our infant son. Any sane person would have seen at a glance that I was stretched way too thin, but I thought I could "do it all," and for nearly two years, I tried to. I worked nonstop, was stressed out virtually all the time, and wasn't sleeping well. My body had started breaking down—and I was only in my early thirties!

After our second son was born, I took two weeks off to be at home. This period of unexpected rest shocked me. Suddenly I realized how normal it had become for me to feel stressed, exhausted, and depleted. As soon as I returned to work, I resigned from my administrative duties and returned to "just" being a physician (and a parent). I still welcomed the challenge of long, vigorous days at work—but I also welcomed the corresponding time of "just being." Instead of turning myself into a perpetual-motion machine, I was finally getting in touch with my body's and spirit's need for a *cycle* that alternated naturally between work and rest.

Let me be very clear: Stress itself—the need to work hard, a set of challenges, a busy day, or even a busy month—is not the problem. The problem comes when we experience our daily demands as unceasing, when the demands never let up, when our lives have become one endless round of activity with no relaxation. To alter this literally depressing pattern, we must slow down and honor our body's need for balance.

Our bodies are governed by larger cycles as well. Most significant to our daily rhythm is a set of brief cycles known as *ultradian rhythms*. During the first ninety minutes or so of each cycle, we feel alert, focused, creative, and productive. But then the natural "rest period" follows, and for about fifteen to twenty minutes, we feel increasingly fatigued, bored, "foggy," or sad. Our body is geared up for activity during that first hour and a half, but then it needs a break.

Although taking a break may seem impossible to those of us with busy schedules, honoring our body's need for rest actually makes us *more* productive. Not only do we get more work done during the day, we also end each day feeling less stressed, more energized, and happier.

So start noticing when you need a break, paying attention to such signals as a yawn, the feeling of muscle fatigue, the need to stretch, or the loss of focus—making silly mistakes, forgetting simple things, or daydreaming. You might simply notice that the workday feels harder, a situation seems more tense, or you feel unproductive. Either way, take a break, as little as a moment or two to alter your breathing; as much as twenty minutes to take a walk, listen to music, or do a short set of stretches. Your goal is to have no goal—but simply to be aware of yourself and your body.

♂〰〰♀

Calming Activities

Choose these when you're feeling restless, anxious, or inattentive. These are especially helpful for people with serotonin-deficient depression.

- Try the Calming Breath Technique, described above.
- Eat a small serotonin-boosting snack like fruit, yogurt, or a granola bar (see Chapter 4).
- Drink some filtered or spring water or some unsweetened juice—but no caffeine.
- Go for a slow, pleasant walk in which you allow yourself to focus on your body and your environment, leaving behind your thoughts

and preoccupations (for more suggestions on walking as relaxation, see the "Walking Meditation" described in Chapter 15).

- Massage your neck, shoulders, or feet. (In the ideal world, you'd have a friend or loved one do this for you, but self-massage can also be pleasant and relaxing.)
- Spend five to ten minutes stretching.
- Sit and meditate for five to ten minutes, focusing on your breathing. You can simply sit and allow yourself to focus on the breath, or you can follow my suggestions for meditation in Chapter 15.
- Just sit quietly or lie down, focusing your attention on soft music or nature sounds—or on nothing at all.

Energizing Activities

Choose these when you're feeling tired, sluggish, or dull. These are especially helpful for people with norepinephrine/dopamine– deficient depression.

- Try the Energizing Breath Technique, described above.
- Eat a small dopamine-boosting snack, such as cheese, nuts, or a high-protein bar (see Chapter 4).
- Drink some filtered or spring water, unsweetened juice, or green tea. Avoid coffee, especially after twelve noon.
- Go for a brisk walk or take some other form of vigorous exercise.
- Do some energizing yoga postures.
- Do some tai chi, qigong, or other form of meditative movement.
- Simply move your body—walk, stretch, or do a few simple calisthenics—in whatever way feels good in that moment.

CHARTING THE RHYTHMS OF YOUR DAY

Beyond the two-hour ultradian rhythms, our lives are also set to the *circadian* or *diurnal* rhythm of the daily cycle that regulates sleep and wakefulness. In fact, our biological clock is set not to a twenty-four-hour day but to one that lasts closer to twenty-five hours. Presumably that gap between nature's clock and our body's internal sense of timing gave primitive humans some flexibility with regard to when they slept and woke, enabling them to stay up all night if survival required it. Ideally, though, we use the daily cues of the sun's rising and setting—and of our own regular sleep and wake times—to reset our inner clocks each day to a twenty-four-hour cycle.

Our daily clock is set by the pineal gland, which releases a hormone known as melatonin—ideally at the same time each evening, preparing us for sleep. Likewise, our adrenal hormones, including the stimulating hormones of cortisol and adrenaline, are released at particular times throughout the day. Ideally, as night turns into morning, the adrenal gland releases more hormones, bringing us out of the deeper stages of sleep and preparing us to take on the day. Our adrenal levels rise throughout the morning, peaking around noon, so that for most of us, morning is our most productive time. Our cortisol drops in mid- to late afternoon—a time when many of us might benefit from a short nap—and then rises during the early part of the evening. As night draws near, our adrenal hormones drop once again, preparing us to rest and sleep. When the cycle works as it should, our adrenal hormones are at the low point during the early to middle part of our sleep cycle, coinciding with our period of deepest sleep.

As you can see, the ups and downs of our adrenal hormones—also known as stress hormones—mirror an ideal workday, with periods of intense activity alternating with times of rest. But if we're constantly busy, worried, or preoccupied, we never give our bodies a chance to recharge, and both our adrenals and our entire body suffer as a result. Moreover, if, like so many of us, we've taught ourselves to ignore our body's cries for rest, relaxation, and "downtime," we lose the ability to give ourselves what we need. Our depleted adrenal system becomes unable to release the stimulating hormones we need to provoke us to maximum activity, and we feel tired, dragged out, and, frequently, depressed. I believe that under such circumstances, our brain chemistry actually alters, so that depression recurs more and more frequently in response to fewer and less severe triggers. In my opinion, the gradual and continual depletion brought on by unremitting stress and the failure to honor our body's need for rest is a major factor in both the onset and the recurrence of depression.

Your Brain-Healthy Daily Cycle: Aligning with Nature Through Circadian Rhythms

- Remember that it is normal and healthy to have ups and downs throughout the day. Don't try to plow through them or to push yourself to sustained levels of activity; instead, maximize your productivity as well as your health by working with your natural rhythms, not against them.
- The first few hours of sleep are the deepest, making this the most important time for healing and tissue repair.
- Stress hormones, levels of alertness, organ function, and body temperature reach their lowest points around 3 to 4 a.m., so ideally, you will be sleeping deeply at this hour. The body needs deep sleep to heal itself, as evidenced by the fact that conditions that are associated with a lot of pain or poor healing, such as fibromyalgia, are linked to poor sleep—and poor serotonin levels. Ensuring that you get a lot of deep, healing sleep is key to both recovering from depression and to preventing another episode.
- For most of us, it is best to arise between 6 a.m. and 8 a.m., because this keeps us in sync with nature's rhythms, which are largely dictated by sunrise and sunset. If we fall too far out of alignment with nature, most of us won't feel quite as good. You'd be surprised at how much your energy, focus, and productivity are affected by the degree of regularity in your sleep/wake times.
- Given our natural cycle of stress hormones, mornings tends to be our most productive and alert time of day. For most of us, this is a good time for creative work or problem solving.
- If you can, try to take a twenty- to thirty-minute nap shortly after lunch. This is a low point for most of us, and a short nap before 3 p.m. can be rejuvenating.
- Midafternoon is often another productive time for most of us.
- Late afternoon—from 4 p.m. to 7 p.m.—is the time when most of us begin to shift from activity to inactivity. Whatever your daily schedule, start to notice how your biorhythms change over the course of the day, and begin to work with them rather than to override them, remembering that the more regular your schedule, the healthier your brain is likely to be.
- In the late evening hours—9 p.m. to 11 p.m.—the body needs to pre-

pare for sleep. Try not to work or be very active during the final one to two hours before you head off to bed.

SLEEP: YOU CAN'T LIVE (WELL) WITHOUT IT

We've learned to ignore not only our daytime cycles but our nightly needs as well. Before electricity was widely available, our sleep schedules were largely tied to sunrise and sunset, and people's sleep averaged over nine hours per night. By the middle of the twentieth century, the average sleep time was closer to eight hours, and now it's down to seven or less—with disastrous results for our brain chemistry. I work a lot with college students whose typical bedtime is 2 a.m. or 3 a.m., with a total sleep time of only four to six hours per night. On the weekends, they may sleep longer, which further throws off their biorhythms. If you're young and resilient, you may be able to shake off the problems caused by these irregular rhythms. But if you're prone to a mood or anxiety problem, you simply *cannot* feel good if you live like this.

After diet and exercise—which can also help improve sleep—getting adequate sleep is the most important thing you can do to overcome depression. If you're suffering from temporary or chronic insomnia—the inability to fall asleep or stay asleep—you may already realize how crucial sleep is to improving your mood. You may need to take some extra steps to help yourself sleep more regularly and continuously. Or you may simply need to work a bit harder at maintaining a regular sleep schedule. Either way, follow these suggestions for a month and see how much your brain chemistry improves with regular, healthful sleep.

Your Brain-Healthy Sleep Plan: Sleeping for Better Brain Chemistry
- **Get as much sleep as you need.** The vast majority of Americans are relatively sleep-deprived. Most studies suggest that the average adult requires around eight hours, though your own need for sleep may lie within a range of seven to nine hours. And while seniors don't sleep as well as they age, they still need about as much sleep as they did when they were younger. The average person probably gets about an hour less sleep than he or she needs.

- *Know how much sleep you need.* Here's a good way to find out your ideal amount of sleep. Pick a wake-up hour and stick to it for a few weeks, using an alarm clock if necessary. Begin the experiment by going to bed at your current bedtime. Then, every couple of days, go to bed ten or fifteen minutes earlier. Keep adding sleep until you wake up naturally, without an alarm. You'll need to give this experiment a few weeks, but when you are waking regularly on your own, you're probably getting the sleep you need.

- *Have a comfortable bedroom.* Keep your sleep chamber cool, dark, and well insulated against sound. A good mattress is a smart investment. A source of white noise can help if night noises—including a spouse's snoring—wake you up.

- *Develop positive associations with bedtime.* Go into your bedroom only for sleep and sex—and lie down to sleep only when you already feel sleepy. If you can't fall asleep within fifteen minutes, leave your bedroom and engage in a quiet, calming activity until you feel sleepy again. Stay away from TV and the computer, both of which emit stimulating rays of light that will interfere with your sleep cycle.

- *Avoid stimulants and alcohol.* Even if you drink your tea or coffee before noon, it can affect your nightly sleep. So can the caffeine in some medications, including aspirin and other pain relievers, the nicotine in tobacco, the decongestants in cough or cold remedies, and herbal products containing ma huang, guarana, or yerba maté. Even chocolate is mildly stimulating. And while a glass of wine before bed may be relaxing, having more than one or two drinks can interfere with your sleep quality, particularly if you tend toward waking early in the morning or in the middle of the night.

- *Eat right for your sleep needs.* If you've got temporary or chronic insomnia, you're probably low in serotonin. Follow the serotonin-enhancing diet described in Chapter 4, eat lightly in the evenings, and limit foods high in protein and fat in the evenings. Also, don't eat really spicy food in the evening—the extra work involved in digesting may keep you awake.

- *Eat a bedtime snack.* A healthy carb snack an hour before bedtime can ease the strain of fasting overnight, while high-serotonin food can help you sleep. Try a tryptophan-rich food such as milk, fruit (banana or pineapple), nuts (almonds or walnuts), a little cereal, whole-grain bread, or brown rice.

- **Use heat.** We fall asleep most easily when the body is cooling off, so about an hour before your bedtime, take a warm bath, perhaps with some aromatherapy oils. Keep your bedroom cool, using plenty of covers to keep yourself warm.

- **Exercise.** Remember, one of the great benefits of exercise is improved sleep. A study of elderly patients published in the *Journal of the American Medical Association* in 1997 showed that when they engaged in walking and other low-impact aerobics for just four days a week, they enjoyed an hour more sleep each night.[6] Exercise is especially helpful if you're suffering from insomnia related to stress, anxiety, or muscle tension. Don't exercise right before bed, however. Exercise warms you up and energizes you, so ideally you'll do it mid- to late afternoon.

- **Develop a calming bedtime routine.** Avoid stimulating activities like picking up the house, watching TV, or working on your computer during the hour before bedtime. Instead, try reading, listening to quiet music, meditating, or using the Calming Breath Technique described above.

- **Keep a regular sleep schedule.** One of the most common reasons for being unable to fall asleep is getting out of your proper biorhythm, usually by staying up late and then sleeping late the next morning. The next night, you're not ready to fall asleep at your usual time, and sleep problems begin. I recommend getting up at roughly the same time each day, no matter when you go to bed. Make up for short nights with a brief nap or an earlier bedtime. Particularly if you are having trouble sleeping, I strongly recommend sticking to the same wake-up time every day, even on weekends and holidays. Varying your wake-up time by more than an hour or so means you probably won't feel as well.

- **Use naps properly.** Naps are usually a healthy and stress-relieving practice. But if you have insomnia, avoid naps until you can sleep through the night—no matter how tired you get. If you're not concerned about insomnia, stick to twenty- to forty-five-minute naps in the middle of the day. If your bedtime is 11 p.m., for instance, you should restrict naps to the time between noon and 3 p.m., or you might have trouble falling asleep.

- **Keep a sleep log.** Of course you don't need to keep a log if you're not having trouble sleeping. But if you suffer from insomnia, note your bedtime, wake-up time, what you do before bed each evening, what you eat each night, and how well rested you feel the following day. Then look for patterns and clues about what might be causing your insomnia. Obsessive thoughts? A heavy meal? A habit of working on the bills just before bedtime? Experiment with changing patterns that don't work while following the other recommendations on this list.

- **Consider acupuncture.** Many people who have trouble sleeping report good results for insomnia.

HERBS AND SUPPLEMENTS FOR SLEEP

Note: Take any type of sleep aid—include snacks, supplements, and medication—from half an hour to an hour before bedtime.

- **Consider taking B vitamins, calcium, and/or 5-HTP to help you sleep.** For more information, see Chapter 5.
- **Melatonin: 1 to 3 mg (although some use as little as 0.3 mg).** I recommend the sublingual form, which is placed under the tongue and gets absorbed faster and better than if it is taken by mouth. This hormone is produced by the pineal gland to help set the timing of sleep's onset. Normally, we release more melatonin automatically as the sky grows dark, but those of us who've trained ourselves to stay up late may need some help resetting our daily clocks. That "second wind" you get after you've stayed up past your normal bedtime is the effect of melatonin wearing off, since it's only good for an hour or two. If you're having trouble staying asleep, melatonin probably won't help you, but it can make it easier for you to fall asleep, particularly if you need help resetting your biological clock after jet lag, shift work, or when you've gotten into the habit of staying up too late. For these problems, taking melatonin for just a few days should suffice. I don't usually recommend using a melatonin supplement long-term: We haven't studied its effects for a long enough time, and the supplement may also suppress mood and sexual function. But longer-term use in the dosage that I've recommended should be safe and helpful for the elderly who suffer from a sleep disturbance or for adults who have "delayed sleep phase syndrome," a condition in which you have ongoing difficulty falling asleep on time and then can't get up in the morning. This syndrome is a fairly common pattern in people with irregular schedules or those who suffer from seasonal affective disorder (SAD).
- **Valerian root: 50–200 mg three times a day for anxiety, 300–900 mg**

for sleep (freeze-dried extract standardized to 0.8 percent valeric acid). For sleep, take an hour or so before bed.

Before the development of barbiturates, valerian was the mainstay sedative in Europe and America. A great deal of literature exists, especially in Germany, on its effectiveness in preventing anxiety, and there's good evidence for believing that it improves sleep onset and quality.[7] Note that it may take two to three weeks to become effective. I believe valerian is quite safe, but it does depress the central nervous system, so don't take valerian after you've been drinking, smoking marijuana, or consuming any other depressant. It may also enhance the effects of anesthetics, so don't take it the night before surgery. It appears safe even for long-term use, but I generally recommend taking a break from herbal therapies every few months.[8]

Natural Ways to Raise Your Melatonin Levels

- Eat fewer calories.
- Eat fish once or twice a week.
- Increase magnesium intake.
- Exercise.
- Avoid alcohol.

FOLLOWING THE CYCLE OF THE SEASONS: WORKING WITH WINTER

Cindy was like many people in my rural Minnesota town, who welcome winter with decidedly mixed feelings. Even during the warmer months, Cindy tended to be sluggish, overweight, and low energy, which suggested that her system lacked stimulation. As the winter set in, she tended to sleep more heavily and for longer hours, and she often found it difficult to wake up in the morning.

Cindy suffered from seasonal depression—known as seasonal affective disorder or SAD. SAD is a condition that affects many of us living in the North: a type of depression that seems to result from a shortage of daylight. SAD may affect as many as 10 million Americans each year, usually between late October and March, though some people notice their mood change as early as September and don't feel better until

May. SAD is also four times more common in women than in men, per-haps because the female hormones of estrogen and progesterone are af-fected by light and melatonin levels.

The brain uses serotonin molecules to make melatonin. So if in-creased darkness leads to a rise in melatonin production, your serotonin levels are likely to suffer. At the same time, a lack of exercise, an over-consumption of refined carbs, sweets, and "comfort foods," and excessive sleep may have contributed to a dopamine/norepinephrine deficiency. So typically, people with SAD experience both the carbohydrate crav-ings associated with low serotonin levels and the weight gain, stress sen-sitivity, and sluggishness that accompany norepi/dopa shortages.

Certainly Cindy struggled a great deal with SAD, feeling heavy and mentally slow for much of the winter. She described her condition as like "moving through molasses," and she reported getting sleepy every evening within an hour or two after the sun had set. Other people with SAD resist this pull toward an early bedtime, catching a second wind later that night and routinely staying up too late. Both SAD patients who go to bed early and those who stay up late tend to have trouble get-ting out of bed in the morning, particularly if they have to wake up be-fore sunrise.

For Cindy, as for other SAD patients, I recommended measures to improve serotonin levels, regulate circadian rhythms, and increase en-ergy and movement. Although some people need medication when they're first diagnosed with SAD, Cindy was able to overcome this syn-drome with nonmedical means. From October through April, she used a light box to give herself phototherapy early in the morning and late in the afternoon. (For more on phototherapy, see below.) She also followed my recommendation to establish a daily routine emphasizing regularity, less sleep, and an earlier rising time. She began a fairly heavy exercise routine, including circuit (weight) training three days a week and run-ning another two or three days per week, and she made regular use of my Energizing Breathing Technique. Finally, she ate more protein with every meal, reduced her percentage of calories from carbohydrates, and ate lighter foods, as one might do in the heat of the summer—salads, water-filled fruits, low-fat foods, fish, and lean meats. She supplemented her diet with B-complex vitamins, fish-oil capsules, and 500 mg of DL-phenylalanine three times daily.

After a few weeks, Cindy felt considerably lighter, was more energetic and alert, and needed less sleep. She was also losing a bit of weight, which pleased her. But she continued to have a flat, low mood and a fairly passive approach to her life. Ultimately, she needed to adopt both the Ayurvedic techniques for her Earth/kapha type and the Buddhist psychological approaches for her "Denial" or "Confusion" emotional type (see Steps Two and Three). Meanwhile, though, Cindy had successfully overcome the seasonal aspect of her depression without medication.

Even my patients who do need medication are usually able to prevent further recurrence of SAD once they know how to eat, exercise, and use phototherapy as the winter draws in. Significantly, the treatment I recommended for Cindy is also useful for nonseasonal depression, PMS, and bulimia, while symptoms that respond to light therapy include excessive sleep and appetite, bingeing on high carbohydrate foods, irritability, decreased libido, poor concentration, and lack of energy.

RESPONDING TO SAD: LIGHT THERAPY OR PHOTOTHERAPY

When bright light at the level of 2,500 lux or more enters the eyes, it raises serotonin and perhaps also dopamine levels, and it can also help normalize circadian rhythms. A light box is a worthwhile investment. Most use full-spectrum light of 10,000 lux, with filters to take out UV radiation. Some can be purchased now for about two hundred to three hundred dollars. (See Appendix C, Resources.)

Since you're trying to trick your brain into thinking that the sun is rising earlier and setting later than it is, light therapy is best done between 6 a.m. and 9 a.m., and from 4 p.m. to 7 p.m. Don't practice it too close to bedtime—it might keep you awake. Generally, the best time for light therapy is thirty to sixty minutes in the morning, just after waking, but if you're finding yourself feeling sleepy much earlier than your normal bedtime or if your morning routine doesn't leave time for light therapy, you can do all or part of the exposure in the late afternoon or *early* evening. Some of my patients have had great results with a twenty- to thirty-minute exposure twice a day.

- Use light at an intensity of 5,000 lux to 10,000 lux. Full-spectrum light is best but not essential. Use a UV filter to protect your skin.

- Sit close to the light, within eighteen to twenty-four inches, with your eyes open. You don't have to look directly at the light, and it's fine for you to read or do anything else that keeps you close to the light.
  - Reduce your exposure if you experience such side effects as eye irritation, an agitated or euphoric mood, or sleep disturbance. You shouldn't have to discontinue treatment, just adjust it a bit.
  - A healthy carbohydrate snack, combined with a little protein, eaten mid- to late afternoon, may make phototherapy more effective.
  - Exercise also makes light therapy more effective.

RESPONDING TO SAD: DAWN SIMULATION

If you just can't get out of bed as early as I'm recommending, try a dawn simulator—a bright light attached to a clock and a rheostat. Set the time you want to wake up, and the light comes on very gradually about a half hour before. The light in your room gradually increases, and you'll wake when your room is bright enough. The idea is to mimic a natural sunrise, a process that might have similar benefits to the light box. If the light doesn't wake you up, an alarm helps finish the job. (See Appendix C, Resources.)

Combining the light-box treatment and the dawn simulator will have the most powerful effect on your SAD. The next most effective intervention is the light alone, and then the dawn simulator alone. I like telling my patients about the dawn simulator because, after the initial purchase, it requires no time or effort and can really help with the sleep phase disorder. So for people who can't sit in front of the light box, it's a great option.

Responding to SAD: Some Natural Options

- Increase your exposure to natural light.
- Follow the serotonin-enchancing diet, but with fewer carbohydrates overall and a focus on complex rather than simple carbs. However, if you feel sluggish, you should do the opposite: Add more protein to your

diet and follow the norepinephrine-enhancing diet. I like to tell my patients to eat the way they naturally would in the summer: light, water-rich foods like salads and fruits, and fewer overall calories.

- Exercise more, and more vigorously.
- Sleep less overall, and make a significant effort to get up at the same time each day, preferably before 8 a.m.
- Add supplements to your diet. With so little exposure to sunlight in winter, our bodies may become relatively deficient in vitamin D. Some studies have shown benefit from adding vitamin D to the diet of SAD sufferers, so try adding 600 mg to 1000 mg of vitamin D_3 to your daily diet during the winter. Also take B-complex vitamins and essential fatty acids as described in Chapter 5.

HYPERSOMNIA: TOO MUCH OF A GOOD THING

During the winter, Cindy suffered from hypersomnia, the condition of getting too much sleep. Hypersomnia is a common side effect of both SAD and norepi/dopa-deficient depression, as well as a problem that plagues people with an irregular sleep routine. If you're struggling with hypersomnia, you'll sleep ten to twelve hours in a single day, but feel more depressed and less rested as a result, especially if the pattern continues for several days. Hypersomnia usually lasts for several days—but even a single day of too much sleep can leave you feeling sluggish and depressed, besides shifting your sleep-wake cycle and interfering with a regular schedule.

Your mood and energy may improve significantly if you restrict your sleep to eight hours a night and get up by 8 a.m. or even earlier. If you think you're suffering from hypersomnia—where you routinely sleep excessively as opposed to just a day or two of "catching up"—try the norepinephrine-enhancing diet in Chapter 4, get more vigorous exercise, and practice the Energizing Breath Technique described above.

FOLLOWING THE CYCLE OF THE SEASONS: SPRING CLEANING

After the winter comes the spring, and after the drawing-in time of darkness comes the season for cleansing and detoxifying. Give your body a spring cleaning with a detoxification program that allows you to shed all the poisons that accumulate from our polluted air and water, as well as from all the food additives, chemicals, pesticides, and hormones in our food and the toxins in our cleaning products, insect sprays, deodorizers, perfumes, paints, and exhaust fumes, not to mention the chemical odors of plastics, adhesives, and other artificial products. While only some of us have developed a marked environmental sensitivity to one or more of these assaults, virtually all of us suffer from a kind of low-grade toxicity that can—without our even being aware of it—affect not only our health but our brain chemistry and our mood. I believe that subtle toxic exposure plays a role in the onset of mood disorders and should be part of what we address in a holistic treatment approach.

Even though I live in a rural area, far from the auto and industrial pollution of a large city, I know that I and my patients are still at risk from the chemicals used to fertilize our fields and keep our crops insect-free. And when my patients—both rural and urban—have tried to overcome their chemical sensitivity by completely avoiding toxins, I've seen it limit their lives to an unacceptable degree. (I think it's smart to try to avoid toxins, but not to get compulsive about it.)

Still, if we can't rule toxins out of our environment entirely, at least we can minimize our risk in order to keep our brains and bodies functioning as well as possible. For example, we can buy organic foods, especially meat and diary, and we can purchase earth-friendly—and brain-friendly—cleaning products, paints, carpeting, and other household products, even as we avoid perfume, cologne, and deodorizers. But beyond reducing our exposure, we need to take measures to strengthen and cleanse our bodies. Here are some suggestions for cleansing, detoxifying, and protecting yourself from the cell damage that can occur from exposure to toxins.

**Your Brain-Healthy Detox Plan: Ridding Yourself of Toxins
for Better Brain Chemistry**

- Breathe—practice deep, cleansing breathing to rid your body of unwanted chemicals.
- Clean your air ducts, grow indoor plants, and get a good air filter to purify your indoor air. Look for a HEPA filter and/or an ionizing air cleaner.
- Drink lots of pure water—a minimum of six to eight eight-ounce glasses a day. Start the day with two to four glasses of water just after arising. Be sure that the water itself is pure so that you aren't adding toxins by drinking it. I recommend carbon-filtered water. Distilled water or water treated with a reverse-osmosis filter is more likely to be pure.
- Eat organic foods as much as possible.
- Get plenty of antioxidants into your diet, as they help protect cells from the damage of free radicals. Eat the antioxidant-rich foods listed in Chapter 4 and follow the antioxidant supplement regimen suggested in Chapter 5.
- Sweat—exercise and heat therapies like saunas and steam rooms help rid the body of toxic buildup.
- Use nontoxic, earth- and brain-friendly cleansers in the home and office.
- Buy natural soaps, lotions, and shampoos, and avoid perfume or cologne.
- Consider an occasional detoxifying regimen, perhaps with a period of fasting. I like doing a spring detox sometime in April and another in the fall, to prepare for winter.

Your Detox Regimen

I recommend undertaking this regimen twice a year, in April and October—as the seasons turn. I myself do this twice-yearly detox, and it always leaves me feeling lighter and more energized.

- For three to seven days, eat only the following cleansing foods:
  - steamed or fresh vegetables, especially green leafy vegetables
  - fresh fruits, especially berry and citrus fruits; grapefruit is especially helpful

- a little protein—a boiled egg or a bit of fish or chicken—if you're feeling fatigued
- make a vegetable broth by cooking a variety of organic vegetables for a couple of hours in a large quantity of water; drink this in between meals whenever hungry

• For the entire month, including the days on the detox diet, you may take an herbal cleansing supplement both for the colon and the body in general. There are many good products on the market, and they are available in health-food stores or at holistic practitioners' offices.
• Your detox month is a good time to take a sauna or a steam bath a few times per week.

STEP TWO:

Know Your Ayurvedic Type

7

AYURVEDIC WISDOM: WHICH TYPE ARE YOU?

To supplement my understanding of Western brain chemistry, I've found it extremely useful to draw upon the centuries-old healing system from India known as Ayurveda, "the science of life." A comprehensive and time-tested approach to health and wellness, Ayurvedic medicine may well be the oldest system of healing in the world. It is still widely practiced in India, as well as among some practitioners in this country, including the famed holistic physician Deepak Chopra, from whom I've learned what I know about this Mind-Body medicine.

While I'm not an Ayurvedic practitioner myself, I appreciate Ayurveda's integration of body, mind, and spirit and its vision of health as balance and harmony. I also find Ayurveda's system of categorizing different constitutional types very useful in understanding depression, particularly since, as we've seen, the imbalances associated with each type resemble the neurotransmitter imbalances I described in Step One. Learning your Ayurvedic type is your first step toward crafting antidepression strategies specifically tailored to suit your own personal body, mind, and spirit.

IDENTIFY YOUR AYURVEDIC TYPE

Ayurveda describes three major mind-body types, or *doshas*. Each dosha is a specific type of energy, and all of us possess some of each—but in different proportions.

Besides corresponding to Western brain-chemical types, Ayurvedic categories also resemble Western body types: ectomorphs (thin, wiry build), mesomorphs (muscular, strong build), and endomorphs (fleshy, heavy build). In Ayurveda, though, each physical category is linked to mental and psychological patterns, as well as habits and lifestyle.

Find out which Ayurvedic type you are by taking the following questionnaire. For each question, circle the answer that best describes you. If more than one answer seems to fit, circle both, or all three:

1. Normally, my body is:
   a. thin and light
   b. of medium build and muscular
   c. solid and large-boned

2. My skin tends to be:
   a. dry, cool, or rough
   b. soft, warm, or splotchy
   c. thick, smooth, or oily

3. I have the most trouble tolerating weather that is:
   a. cold
   b. hot
   c. cool and damp

4. My hair is best described as:
   a. dry, curly, thin
   b. fine, straight, may have early balding or graying
   c. thick, wavy, oily

5. My appetite tends to be:
   a. variable and irregular
   b. strong, occasionally excessive
   c. steady, and I gain weight easily

6. Skipping meals is:
   a. something that happens because of my erratic schedule and appetite
   b. hard for me, making me crabby or irritable
   c. easy for me

7. My bowel habits are:
   a. irregular, often constipated or dry stools

b. regular, frequent, often loose stools
c. regular, often oily stools

8. My physical activity level tends to be:
   a. high, often restless
   b. medium, often driven
   c. low, often lethargic

9. My movements are usually:
   a. quick, random
   b. strong, purposeful
   c. slow, methodical

10. My mind is best described as:
    a. quick, active, restless
    b. sharp, intelligent, critical
    c. calm, slow, thoughtful

11. I tend to learn:
    a. quickly
    b. determinedly
    c. slowly

12. My memory is usually:
    a. good for short term, poor for long term
    b. strong and detail-oriented
    c. slow to develop but with good retention

13. My sleep tends to be:
    a. light and easily disrupted
    b. sound, needing less than others
    c. deep, needing more than others

14. When emotionally balanced, I tend to be:
    a. lively, creative, and enthusiastic
    b. determined, friendly, and successful
    c. calm, sweet-natured, and easygoing

15. When stressed, I easily become:
    a. anxious, insecure, or moody

b. irritable, impatient, or critical
c. sluggish, complacent, or overly attached

SCORING: Count the number of answers that were:
   a:_____ (this corresponds to vata, or Air type)
   b:_____ (this corresponds to pitta, or Fire type)
   c:_____ (this corresponds to kapha, or Earth type)

If you scored significantly higher in one category, that's your type. If you've got high scores in two categories, you're a combination type. If you've got relatively equal scores in all three categories, you're that rare phenomenon, a three-part combination type.

In the rest of this chapter and the following three, you'll learn more about each of the three Ayurvedic types. I urge you to read about all three types, even if you fit one type very strongly. Although each of us is dominated by the energy associated with our type—Air, Fire, or Earth—we each have elements of all three energies within us. So while you're most likely to go "out of balance" in your dominant energy, you might experience other kinds of imbalances as well. Reading through all three chapters will give you the best overview of an Ayurvedic perspective so you can apply it to your own situation with more flexibility rather than pigeonholing yourself into a single type.

This perspective, too, corresponds to Western biochemistry. Although people tend to fall into certain patterns, with the same chemicals coming up short each time, we all experience individual variations. A person who is normally sluggish might suddenly become anxious or agitated because of an unexpected shift in brain chemistry that was caused by changes in diet, stress, or some other factor. In Western terms, we'd talk about levels of dopamine and norepinephrine. In Ayurveda, we might talk about imbalances in your Fire energy. So even if you are normally a sluggish Earth type, you will need to know what an angry Fire imbalance looks like.

Knowing about all three types is especially important if you're a combination type, who scored fairly evenly on two or even three of the categories. If that is the case, you need to follow the recommendations for both or all of your types. If the recommendations conflict, use your intuition and a little experimentation to see which path to follow. An Ayurvedic practitioner can also help you fine-tune your approach.

By the way, I myself am a combination type, both vata/Air and pitta/Fire. When I'm living a life of balance, I enjoy many of the good qualities of both types. When I get stressed or out of balance, I tend to fall into the problematic patterns of both.

VATA: LIGHT, QUICK, AND CHANGEABLE AS AIR

Body-Mind Traits

- body tends to be light and thin
- skin and hair are often dry
- hands and feet get cold easily
- movements are quick, and may seem random or scattered
- appetite is quite variable
- craves sweet, sour, and salty tastes
- prefers hot drinks
- bowel habits are irregular
- sleep is light and easily disrupted
- daily routine tends to be inconsistent, as in bedtime, wake-up time, mealtime

Vata in Balance

- mind is active, creative, and full of ideas
- fast learner (although tends to forget quickly)
- tends to be enthusiastic and energetic, often excelling at initiating new things
- often lively, fun, and a good conversational partner

Vata Under Stress

- becomes constipated
- has a restless mind
- allows his/her routine to become scattered and erratic
- grows fearful, nervous, and has trouble sleeping
- is prone to an anxious depression

Robert: A Story of Vata Imbalance

Robert is a young law student. While still an undergraduate, he'd excelled in school, taking easily to nearly every subject. In fact, he liked so many different courses, he had a hard time deciding what to major in and finally settled on law only because it left open so many possibilities for careers.

Robert had never really been depressed. Nor had he really begun to struggle until he started law school. The demands it made on his time left little room for pursuing his many interests. He became stressed, and he started to doubt both his abilities and his choice of career. Suddenly Robert felt insecure, as if he never quite measured up to others. His digestion was unsteady, as were his bowels. His appetite was poor, and he lost weight. He came to rely on caffeine and sugary foods to keep his energy up, and as a result, he became almost constantly tense and anxious. He seldom found time for exercise, other than walking rapidly whenever he had someplace to be. Every night, he'd lie awake, ruminating about the events of the day. At age thirty-two, he seemed to be aging faster than he should.

Robert's wife added her voice of concern: "He used to be so full of fun and enthusiasm, always interested in doing something, going out or getting together with friends. Now, even when he's not working, his mind is somewhere else. I feel like he never even listens to me anymore." Clearly, their relationship was strained, adding another layer of stress.

Robert illustrates many of both the positive and negative aspects of an Air-based constitution. Normally, his mind is quick and he easily grasps new concepts. He has many interests, and he always wants to keep his options open. He likes to stay active, and others experience him as lively, fun, and enthusiastic.

However, when Robert's work hours became too long and school standards too exacting, he lost time for his other pursuits and felt stressed and out of balance. Then the less healthy aspects of his constitution emerged: stress, insecurity, changes in bowel habits and appetite, sugar cravings, insomnia, and anxiety. Robert's case illustrates how a vata constitution is all about movement. And when the movement gets out of control, both the body and mind become restless, tense, and caught up in unproductive overactivity.

PITTA: PASSIONATE, DETERMINED, AND INTENSE AS FIRE

Body-Mind Traits

- medium, often muscular build
- hair is fine and thin, skin tends to be reactive
- extremities are usually warm
- movements are strong and purposeful
- appetite is strong and regular
- likes sweet, bitter and astringent tastes
- prefers cold drinks
- bowels are regular or loose
- sleeps soundly, may not need as much sleep as other types
- daily routine tends to be precise

Pitta in Balance

- mind is keen and sharp and often loves a good debate
- insightful, competent, and accomplished
- often athletic
- seen by others as warm, friendly, and engaging
- when coupled with ambition, may like to be leaders

Pitta Under Stress

- mind becomes overly discriminating, critical, or judging
- can develop diarrhea
- easily gets skin flushing or rashes
- may become compulsive in routine
- easily gets angry, irritable, jealous, and judgmental
- may seek power and control
- is prone to an agitated depression

Larry: A Story of Pitta Imbalance

Larry is a middle-aged farmer from rural Minnesota. He is married with two teenage children. Although he's managed to hold on to his farm, he's felt the struggle of the small family farmer, and both he and his wife have had to take jobs in town just to make ends meet. Their children, meanwhile, have shown little interest in farming, which has been a big disappointment to Larry.

Larry is strong and broad-shouldered, a man with lots of energy who's always worked hard without complaint. But his age and hard life were starting to catch up to him, and he developed back problems that both limited his working and kept him up because of the pain. He couldn't afford to hire help, and with his wife working and his kids busy with school activities, Larry felt that all the pressure of the farm had landed squarely on him. He'd always had a temper; now it seemed as if he was always angry, venting his feelings toward his son in the form of criticism and demands that the son was not willing to meet, while his wife began to worry that Larry and his son would come to blows.

Larry's doctor was concerned, meanwhile, because his blood pressure had been consistently elevated. They were having some trouble getting it under control, a particular danger for a man with a family history of heart attacks at a relatively early age.

Larry reveals many traits of a pitta imbalance. Emotionally, this imbalance is revealed through the anger and irritability that so concerned his family. He also appears flushed, has had problems with diarrhea and hemorrhoids, and struggles with high blood pressure, muscle tension, and pain.

KAPHA: STURDY, SOLID, AND STABLE AS EARTH

Body-Mind Traits

- heavier, solid body and large-boned frame
- hair tends to be thicker, with smooth and oily skin
- body temperature remains cool

- movements are slow and methodical
- appetite is steady
- prefers pungent, bitter, and astringent foods
- bowels tend to be regular
- sleeps deeply and longer than others
- tends to be methodical and easygoing in daily routine

Kapha in Balance

- mind is slower but thoughtful and has a good memory
- may be graceful and elegant in movement
- has a calm and easygoing demeanor and people find kapha type easy to be around
- normally tolerant and forgiving
- tends to be very loyal and devoted friends or partners

Kapha Under Stress

- more likely than other types to remain calm under stress
- may become mentally sluggish or plodding
- tends to indulge in emotional eating and may become obese
- can develop feelings of attachment, greed, or envy
- is prone to a lethargic depression

Gretchen: A Story of Kapha Imbalance

Gretchen's biggest concern was her energy. Never ambitious or high achieving, she had nonetheless felt pretty content with her life. She had found happiness in her second marriage, which had produced one daughter who was about to leave home. She and her husband lived in a pleasant suburb, where she worked as an executive secretary for a company she'd been with for more than fifteen years.

Suddenly Gretchen was feeling lethargic and miserable, a condition she didn't understand. She had felt this way once before, in her early twenties, after her first marriage had collapsed. She'd gradually emerged from that low point with the help of some therapy and gone on to create a good life for herself. Now in her forties, she was mired in depression once again, but this time, nothing had gone wrong to explain it.

When she first came to my office, Gretchen acknowledged that she hadn't taken the best care of herself. She had always struggled a bit with her weight, but in the past year she had gained twenty pounds. She used to walk to help keep her weight stable, but now she felt so sluggish and unmotivated that exercise seemed impossible. Worse, she could hardly drag herself out of bed in the morning, and she never felt as if she fully woke up. As a result, she wasn't always able to get to work on time, and when she was at work, she felt inefficient and always behind. She felt mentally dull and generally depressed, unable to muster up the motivation to do anything about her increasingly severe problems. Normally a reliable worker, she had started making silly mistakes, which upset her boss.

Gretchen is a kapha type, normally content, loyal, and easygoing. She tends to be a little slow and plodding at times, but usually this comes across as steadiness and stability, and she can muster a great deal of endurance, stamina, and calmness under stress.

Her recent struggles, though, suggest that her constitution has become imbalanced. When a kapha type gets out of balance, everything tends to slow down. Thus, Gretchen's thinking is dulled, she has gained weight, and she's sleeping way too much.

UNDERSTANDING MIND-BODY IMBALANCE

What causes our bodies and minds to go out of balance? In my view, imbalance has three sources: physical, mental, and spiritual.

Some illnesses begin in the body and then spread to the mind. Diet, exposure to toxins, exercise, lifestyle, routine, even the people who surround you—all of these factors affect your body and its balance. Once that balance is disturbed, your body's imbalance may infect your mind, creating anxiety, anger, or depression.

However, sometimes it's the mind that unbalances the body. When emotions are repressed—stuffed away in the body and mind rather than felt and expressed—they can easily create an imbalance that manifests as a nervous stomach, a weakened heart, or a number of other stress-related illnesses.

We tend not to link spiritual problems with disease, but clearly they, too, are related to depression. People who have no connection to a higher power, a life of the spirit, or a deeper purpose to life than the daily struggle for existence may be more likely than others to fall into existential despair. If you feel truly alone and alienated, and your life seems devoid of meaning, you've got a recipe for depression, usually with a strong component of fear, or vata imbalance.

If you've experienced a tragedy or another type of disillusion, you might feel angry, disenchanted, despairing, bitter, or resentful—toward God, another country or religion, or someone who has hurt or betrayed you. Holding on to these negative emotions for too long can inspire a pitta imbalance, resulting in an erosion of physical and emotional resources.

More commonly, a person's interest in matters of the spirit simply wanes with lack of attention. The individual may not even be aware of the loss, but he or she gradually realizes that there's no longer an animating or creative force in his or her life, bringing on a state of apathy or darkness, like living within a cloud. A person with a kapha disturbance like this may not feel despairing so much as lifeless—another form of depression.

I consider spiritual problems to be the result not only of your relationship with the divine but also of your relationship with yourself. Depression can result when we don't truly know ourselves or when we fail to honor the deepest dictates of our own heart. The soul has its own language and its own designs upon our lives. When we fail to listen to it, or fail to heed what we hear, we set up the conditions for unhappiness. We'll return to these matters of the soul in Step Three.

REGAINING YOUR NATURAL STATE

Even healthy people can get out of balance and show signs of illness, sometimes for no apparent reason. But if you're aware of your loss of balance, you take the symptoms as early-warning signals and seek a return to inner balance and to health. I personally believe that the most important factor in maintaining health is this inner state. Of course we interact with our environment, encountering viruses, bacteria, toxins, and other stressors. But two people might be exposed to the same cold virus and yet only one develops a cold, just as two people can undergo identical stresses while only one becomes depressed. When you agree that your inner state determines how the environment affects you, you're assuming responsibility for maintaining your own health—and taking on the power to do so.

From this point of view, your goal is not so much to relieve specific symptoms, or even to treat a certain disease, but rather to restore your natural state of inner harmony and balance. Chapters 8, 9, and 10 will offer you more information on how balance can be achieved and maintained for each type of energy so that you can begin to create an approach that is specifically tooled to your physical, mental, and spiritual needs. Many tools are available to help create balance, but we'll focus on those that are particularly effective in treating depression:

- removing the cause of the imbalance
- detoxification
- diet
- exercise
- breathing
- lifestyle and daily routine
- climate and seasonal patterns
- herbal therapies
- emotional release
- meditation and spiritual practice

8

CALMING AIR TYPES

My patient Jeff was a thirty-eight-year-old architect blessed with a quick wit and a seemingly endless ability to devour new information and learn new skills. But the downside of his airy nature—changeable, highly mental, and able to move swiftly—was an overactive mind, always on the alert for signs of danger, most of which didn't exist.

In theory, Jeff knew his worries were groundless, but he still couldn't keep himself from worrying, especially at night. If he'd had a stressful day, he might lie awake for as long as two hours, unable to turn off his mind.

Even when Jeff did fall asleep, his rest was shallow and frequently interrupted by spells of wakefulness, sometimes brought on by one of his many tense dreams. Often he'd wake up with a sore jaw from grinding his teeth throughout the night. Jeff told me that he averaged only six fitful hours of sleep—and that during the day, he ran on nervous energy and caffeine. As a result, his hands tended to shake, his jaw was clenched, and he was subject to mild panic attacks—a racing heart, shallow breathing, and the vague but overwhelming feeling that something bad was going to happen.

Jeff had been taking 100 mg of Zoloft daily for more than three years, and frankly, he'd come to hate it. Although it did help him control his anxiety, he'd gained twenty-five pounds, and the extra flesh was readily apparent on his tall, thin frame. He felt not calm, but sedated, and he didn't like his loss of interest in sex and difficulty reaching orgasm—both common side effects of Zoloft.

Besides, even with the Zoloft, Jeff felt burdened by his anxiety. If things went badly for him at work, his social life hit a snag, or he got a worrisome phone call from his wife, he went into a tailspin, sinking rapidly into a gloomy, stressed-out state in which he alternated between high-pitched worrying and the miserable sense that nothing would ever go right again. When I asked him what he did to soothe or calm himself at these times, he looked at me as though I'd inquired whether he knew how to fly. "I just keep worrying until the worry goes away," he told me bleakly.

Jeff had come to me because he was eager to get off the Zoloft, and he'd heard I'd had considerable success in helping patients switch from medications to more natural ways of altering brain chemistry and overcoming depression. "I have to tell you," he said, his long, thin fingers drumming nervously on the arm of the leather chair in my office, "I've tried to get off it before."

Once, he explained, he'd forgotten to take it with him on vacation—"and within a couple of days, I was miserable. I felt sick to my stomach, shaky, moody—I felt like the whole world was spinning around me and I couldn't get a grip." His mood had improved as soon as he'd resumed his normal dosage, but the experience had left him shaken and pessimistic about ever going without the drug again. Still, he had tried a second time to lower his own dosage, reasoning that perhaps a gradual tapering off might work better than going cold turkey. Once again, his anxiety and depression returned with a vengeance, perhaps even more intensely than before he'd first been medicated.

"That's my story," he concluded. "Pretty bleak, huh." Although Jeff had come to me with the specific goal of getting off Zoloft, I could see that he felt defeated before we'd begun.

"Actually, I don't see it that way," I told him. "Your symptoms sound painful, and frustrating, but they're not necessarily a lifelong condition. I see them more as signs of an imbalance. From a Western perspective, you seem to be low on serotonin—a shortage that your medicine compensates for but doesn't correct. And from an Ayurvedic perspective, you've got a vata nature—an airlike set of mental, physical, and spiritual energies—that has gotten seriously out of balance as well. But both your brain chemistry and your vata energy can be brought back into balance, as long as you're willing to make a few changes."

To Jeff, my optimism came as a revelation. He heard it not as wishful thinking or a generic hope, but rather as grounded in my understanding of both brain chemistry and Ayurveda. I didn't see Jeff's condition as a permanent state that would require lifelong medication, but rather as a temporary imbalance that could be corrected. Even though he might have a chronic propensity toward this particular type of imbalance, that meant only that he had to take special care with his diet, exercise, and lifestyle choices, not that he was necessarily doomed to a lifetime on Zoloft.

"If you had heart problems, I'd help you find the diet and exercise you needed to support your heart," I told him. "And if you were born into a family with a genetic tendency to heart disease, I'd stress that you had to be extra careful about what you ate and how you exercised. In your case, we've got to make sure that you understand the lifestyle choices—the types of eating, breathing, sleeping, and exercise—that will improve the health of your brain."

SEEING BRAIN CHEMISTRY THROUGH EASTERN EYES

The first step, I told Jeff, is to understand what can throw vata energies off balance. There were two ways to look at vata disturbances. One is to remember that all of us possess all three types of energy—vata, pitta, and kapha—and that our vata systems are the most prone to imbalance. Just as air is less stable than fire or earth, so are vata energies more easily disturbed than pitta or kapha energies.

Interestingly, the instability of vata energies in Ayurveda corresponds with the Western scientific notion that a serotonin deficiency is the most common problem associated with depression. Just as vata energies can become unbalanced even in pitta and kapha types, so can serotonin become deficient even in people with other types of brain chemical imbalances, such as norepinephrine/dopamine excess or deficiency. So when people have either vata imbalances or serotonin deficiencies, I usually try to treat those first, no matter what other problems they're experiencing.

But while all of us are prone to vata imbalances, such imbalances are most likely among vata types. These Air types are not necessarily more prone to depression—but when they *do* get depressed, that's how they tend to do it: with a Western diagnosis of anxious depression, characterized by all the symptoms Jeff was experiencing—nervousness, sleeplessness, and excessive worry.

ᏳᎷᏝᎧ

Symptoms of Vata Imbalance

- feeling restless and fretful
- feeling anxious and expecting the worst to happen, as if "looking over your shoulder" or "waiting for the bottom to fall out"
- feelings of inadequacy and low self-worth
- trouble sleeping
- irregular appetite
- poor digestion
- cravings for starches and sweets
- impulsiveness
- scattered thinking
- frenetic or compulsive behavior

Factors That Lead to Vata Imbalance

- stresses—even short-term, seemingly minor stresses
- working long, excessive hours
- not giving yourself sufficient breaks and down time
- feeling unappreciated at work or at home
- adding stimulants to the body, such as caffeine, nicotine, or sugar
- overstimulation, such as noise, movement, being too busy, or being overscheduled
- eating too many foods that don't fit your body type, such as raw, cold foods or bitter and astringent tastes
- skipping meals, especially breakfast
- insufficient or poor quality sleep, having a poor bedtime routine, and/or keeping erratic hours
- having an inconsistent schedule generally
- the changing of the seasons
- a cold, dry climate, such as in fall or winter
- going through a major change, even a positive one like a move or marriage
- suffering a recent loss, or not having dealt with a more remote loss
- failure to identify or express feelings of grief, loss, or fear

ᏳᎷᏝᎧ

DRAWING ON TWO TRADITIONS

"I still don't get it," Jeff said when I'd explained the notion of vata imbalance. "If it really is the same thing as serotonin deficiency, why do you need the Ayurvedic stuff? Why not just stick to the Western diagnosis?"

Certainly, the Western vision of brain chemistry had much to offer, I told Jeff. But the Ayurvedic approach extends this scientific view with rich imagery that offers a multidimensional approach to treatment. Doctors who restrict themselves to a purely chemically oriented view limit their treatment options to the very medications from which Jeff was now trying to get free. While these medications might be useful, I believed they should be supplemented with broader and more variegated responses.

"Think of the way air is unsettled when a storm front moves in," I suggested. "In fact, picture a mental storm, with the wind blowing this way and that. Think of the qualities of the wind and the air it stirs: light and moving, cooling and drying. This imagery helps us understand that a vata imbalance calls for qualities that will help calm the storm and balance the wind, therapies to settle the mind while adding warmth, moisture, and substance to the body."

Drawing on Ayurvedic imagery, I explained, pointed the way toward rebalancing both body energies and brain chemistry. It gave both Jeff and me many ways to think about his condition, rather than simply reducing him to a chemical imbalance. This broader range of thought would eventually translate into a broader palette of solutions than simply prescribing antidepressants (even if, in some cases, antidepressants were also needed).

REBALANCING VATA ENERGIES

Because vata energies are the easiest to disrupt, they are also the easiest to rebalance. So if any of us has a vata imbalance—whether we're a vata type or some other type—sometimes all we need is a little patience, a casual attempt to avoid the stressors mentioned on the list above, and an effort not to aggravate matters any further. Just as a storm often blows over, vata imbalances often pass by themselves.

Sometimes, though, you want to move things along faster. And if the imbalance is prolonged or recurs frequently, you might apply some more vigor to overcoming or preventing it. In those cases, here are a few basic steps you can take:

- **Eliminate stimulants:** Reducing the presence of stimulants is probably the single most useful thing you can do to correct a vata imbalance. Start by cutting out caffeine, decongestants, nicotine, and refined sugar. (Although under most circumstances, vata types can tolerate moderate amounts of refined sugar, excessive sugar can overstimulate the delicate vata system, and when vata types are stressed, even a small amount of sugar can tip the balance.)

  Other stimulants are less noticeable and perhaps more difficult to eliminate, but if cutting back on coffee and cigarettes doesn't help, consider a second round of cuts. Too much noise, visual stimulation, or even movement can make it hard for a vata type to remain focused and balanced. I know one sensitive vata type who finds it difficult to digest his food if he eats in a restaurant where the music is too loud. Likewise, if you're having troubles with anxiety, worry, or depression, you might want to avoid loud, fast, music; exciting action movies; or even loud parties crowded with lots of people. Activities and environments that might be perfectly fine under normal circumstances can be too stressful when vata energies are disturbed.

In Jeff's case, we agreed that he'd reduce his caffeine intake, first by switching from coffee to black tea, and then by moving from black to green tea, a beverage that has even less caffeine and offers many healthful antioxidants besides. Jeff began sleeping better just from making that change. The immediate benefits he experienced from giving up caffeine provided him with the positive reinforcement he needed to make more difficult changes.

- **Identify and address stress.** Removing or reducing excessive stimulation is the first line of defense for vata imbalances, but only rarely is such stimulation at the root of the initial problem. Vata-based anxiety and depression is almost always based in some type of stress, and once you know what the stressor is, you're well on your way to addressing the disorder.

  Sometimes it's easy to identify the stress that set off your vata im-

balance. If you had a major life-changing event, including a positive oc-
currence (falling in love, getting a promotion, having a baby), look no
further. Change is stressful, even—perhaps especially—changes we
have sought and worked toward for many years. Or if you're working
extra hard, dealing with an unusual or prolonged set of family issues, or
just haven't had a vacation in a while, chances are that your vata anxiety and depression are caused by the overload.

Sometimes, though, it's harder to identify a vata-imbalancing stress.
Perhaps you're not as happy with some aspect of your work, your family,
or your relationships as you thought, and this buried discomfort is
emerging as a vata imbalance. Maybe you had an unpleasant experience
with a friend or loved one and convinced yourself it didn't matter—only
to find yourself feeling anxious and uneasy "for no reason" a few days
later. Or perhaps you're simply responding to the change of the seasons
or some other normal and expected transition, which is nonetheless
throwing you off balance.

There is a third type of vata imbalance that I see in many of my patients. This is the anxiety or discomfort that results from your own mind
and thoughts. Suppose, for example, everything in your life is going
along fine, and then you have the sudden thought that you might not
have enough money to retire when you had planned. That thought
would cause no problem if you simply let it pass through your consciousness, but what if it lodges into your mind and won't let go? You start to
nurse your worry, and suddenly you can think of little else. You begin to
be driven by the fear of a poverty-stricken old age, a thought that prevents you from falling asleep and troubles your dreams. You start working extra hours to ensure your financial security, feeling driven and
insecure. Soon you're bingeing on junk foods to soothe your worries and
compensate for how bad you feel. That little seed of a thought has created quite a disturbance in your vata energy, a mental and emotional
disturbance that goes on to stress your body, leading to muscle tension,
headaches, and alterations in your weight. If your worry continues
unchecked, your vata disturbance can develop into a more serious problem, such as chronic low-back pain, fibromyalgia, hypertension—or depression.

As a psychotherapist, I help my patients identify and remove their
stressors, such as toxic relationships or toxic thoughts. If taking this ap-

proach to your depression appeals to you, I highly recommend it. Although it can be painful, frightening, and sometimes daunting to undertake a journey of self-discovery and attempt to undo long-established patterns, the rewards are well worth the effort. But whether or not you choose to find a therapist, you always have the option of self-healing. On a physical level, the best thing you can do is follow the Step Two suggestions for your Ayurvedic type or for the type of disturbance you're experiencing. On a mental, emotional, and spiritual level, you can experience a world of benefit from the Buddhist Psychology of Mindfulness described in Step Three.

FEEDING YOUR VATA ENERGIES

If you're suffering from a vata imbalance, take particular care to follow the dietary guidelines I laid out in Chapter 4, with special attention to the suggestions for serotonin-deficiency depression. Sweet, salty, and sour tastes appeal to an unbalanced vata, who are looking for strong, "solid" sensations to balance all that light, windy energy. Sweet and starchy foods also provide immediate—albeit temporary—boosts in serotonin levels, although when blood sugar falls rapidly in response to the sugar high, serotonin levels crash as well. Over the long run, too much sugar and too many refined carbs will lead to serotonin depletion, making the brain-chemical problem worse and worse.

Your Brain-Healthy Vata Diet: How Air Types Need to Eat
- Ideally, you'll have a meal or snack every four to five hours, including some high-quality protein and complex carbs each time you consume food.
- *Never* skip breakfast! You need the protein and complex carbs to ground you, or you risk "flying into the air," unmoored by moodiness, anxiety, and stress, with any random worry able to blow you off course.
- Seek warm, moist, and moderately heavy foods, with healthy fats and solid textures, to balance your light and airy nature. Nuts, with their healthy oils, are a good choice for vata snacks.
- Pay attention to taste, a key aspect of Ayurveda. Focus on foods that are soothing, the comfort foods that you naturally gravitate toward anyway. (See the chart at the end of this chapter.)

- Likewise, reduce or avoid cooling or drying foods, which tend to aggravate Air types—bitter greens, excessively sour foods, or highly spiced meals.
- Ayurveda stresses the need to balance the six tastes it recognizes: sweet, sour, salty, bitter, pungent (spicy), and astringent. So although you're favoring some tastes, try to get a bit of each taste every time you eat. You may be amazed at how much more balanced you feel.
- Eat only when you're hungry and drink only when you're thirsty. Eat smaller portions so that you can follow my other recommendation of a slow, steady supply of food—a meal or a snack every four or five hours that you're awake. I also recommend that you drink very little just before, just after, and during mealtimes, since fluids dilute the digestive enzymes and make your metabolism less efficient. Sipping just a little water while you eat will give you sufficient liquid to aid digestion without diluting your digestive juices.
- Eat with attention. Avoid the temptation to read or watch TV while you're having a meal. Give your attention to the food. Try to discern the different flavors and texture of the food. And when you begin to feel full, stop eating. If you eat slowly and mindfully, you'll be able to feel when you've had enough to eat, and you can then choose to end your meal.
- Choose your drinks with care. You can balance your vata with warm drinks: teas, warm milk, even warm water.
- Eat with the seasons. Staying in sync with seasonal changes can help keep you in balance. Summer, for example, is not the time for hot, spicy foods, which aggravate your pitta energies—your hot, fiery aspects. You don't need any additional heat during the warm summer months, so when the temperature is high, eat light. If you pay attention to your own seasonal clock, summer is probably a time when you are attracted to cooling foods with high water content—salads, fresh fruits, seafood, smaller amounts of meat, and smaller portions generally. Autumn, on the other hand, is the time to gravitate toward vata-pacifying comfort foods—and so nature provides us with the complex carbs of the autumn harvest, such as squash, pumpkins, and sweet potatoes. As the days shorten and grow colder, we often crave warm soups and stews and hearty fall vegetables. But if you've got a vata imbalance or are a vata type, you can use these soothing autumn foods to balance your airy nature all year round.

Your Brain-Healthy Vata Detox: How Air Types Need to Cleanse
Follow the detox suggestions I shared in Chapter 6, with these special suggestions for vata types:

- Air types need to keep their fasting brief, one to three days at most. If you're undertaking a juice fast, choose a sweet juice like grape juice. You might also find it helpful to try a one-day warm-water fast. While you're fasting, you may find it helpful to use spicy herbs, such as pepper, ginger, or curry, to help eliminate toxins and encourage healthy digestion.
- Sweating out the toxins can help cleanse your system. You can sweat through a vigorous workout, or enjoy heat therapies, such as saunas and steam rooms. Moist heat is especially good at soothing your vata nature.
- If you follow the twice-yearly detox month I suggested in Chapter 6, make a point of taking a wet sauna or sitting in the steam room a few times a week. If you have easy access to a sauna or steam room, twenty to thirty minutes once or twice a day would be ideal for air types during their detox.

EXERCISING YOUR VATA NATURE

Exercise was a major aspect in Jeff's ability to reduce his medication and boost his spirits. Previously, Jeff had seen exercise as primarily vigorous, competitive sport—activity that tended to aggravate his vata nature and contribute to his anxiety and stress levels. But for vata types, I explained, it was more important to engage in regular exercise, four or five days per week, ideally with an activity involving a rhythmic or repetitive movement and the chance to be out in nature. I encouraged Jeff to go for brisk half-hour walks, light jogging, and bike rides, all activities that he enjoyed. As his health and spirits improved, he branched out to cross-country skiing in the winter and canoeing on summer weekends, benefiting from the combination of deep breathing, rhythmic movement, and the grounding, balancing experience of contact with earth and water energies.

Your Brain-Healthy Vata Exercise Plan: Activities for Air Types
Check out my suggestions in Chapter 6 for serotonin-building exercise suggestions, supplemented with these additional principles:

- Soothing, repetitive exercise is best for balancing vata. Vigor is less important than rhythmic activity.

- I recommend light aerobic activity for only about twenty to thirty minutes a day. While three to four times a week is your basic minimum, daily exercise is best.
- A moderate-paced walk is the perfect balancing exercise for Air types. Light biking or dancing are also good choices.
- Yoga or simple stretching are good choices for Air types.
- Exercise in a natural setting is particularly soothing for Air types.
- Don't overexert! A vata constitution does not tolerate exercise that is too vigorous. If you push yourself, you might injure or overstimulate yourself, with counterproductive results.
- Golfing, canoeing, biking, and hiking are all good choices for vata types—anything out-of-doors, relaxed, and enjoyable.
- Yoga promotes strength, balance, and flexibility all at once. It is good for Air types because it can be gentle and soothing, stretching muscles and strengthening joints. Choose a teacher and type of yoga that is relaxing and not overly vigorous, and don't go beyond your own limits. "No pain, no gain" has no place in a life of balance, especially for Air types.
- Tai chi is really meditation in motion. It's wonderful for Air types because it engages the body in light, fluid, and calming movement. Some schools focus more on the martial-arts aspect of tai chi; Air types would do well to find a more relaxed and meditative approach.
- Qigong is related to tai chi, a wonderful practice involving breath work, meditation, and energizing movement. Like tai chi, this is a moderately demanding practice that helps calm both body and mind.

BREATHING AND BIORHYTHMS FOR AIR TYPES

Although Jeff showed slow, steady improvement from his improved diet and exercise, he still needed to work on a steady, regular sleep routine. He was staying up too late, then trying to catch up by sleeping late on weekends. His irregular sleep cycle threw off his biorhythms, making it hard for him to feel good. To restore Jeff's balance, I had him follow the sleep suggestions I make in Chapter 6, to keep him in tune with the earth's cycles.

Jeff found it difficult to maintain an early bedtime, but he did his best. Within a few weeks, his sleep had vastly improved, providing him the reinforcement to stay on his new regime. His energy and mood were getting rapidly better, and we were able to reduce his dose of Zoloft to 50 mg after three weeks, and to 25 mg three weeks after that.

Balancing Your Air Energy Through Breathing

Vata types can really benefit from the Calming Breath Technique described in Chapter 6. Alternate nostril breathing is also good for Air types because it reduces overstimulation. Put your thumb and forefinger gently over one nostril, forcing you to breathe through the other. Then switch sides. Continue to switch sides for a few minutes. For example, you'd start by breathing out through your left nostril, while your right nostril is blocked by your thumb. Then breathe in through the left nostril. Block the left nostril in time to exhale, then inhale, through the right side. Continue breathing in this pattern until you feel rebalanced and destressed.

CIRCADIAN RHYTHMS AND VATA ENERGY

Just as Ayurvedic typing matches Western scientific understanding of brain-chemical types, so does the Ayurvedic understanding of circadian rhythms resemble the views of modern science. As we saw in Chapter 6, each period of the day has its own special energy. While Western science sees the day's rhythms in terms of adrenal hormones and other biochemicals, Ayurveda sees the day in terms of the relative activity of our different *doshas*:

- 6 a.m. to 10 a.m.: a time of increased kapha energy, with a slight feeling of heaviness even after a refreshing sleep.
- 10 a.m. to 2 p.m.: Pitta increases. You start feeling hungry, your body becomes warmer, and your mind grows more focused and discerning, making this a good time for mentally demanding work.
- 2 p.m. to 6 p.m.: Vata rises. You feel active and light during this period—a good time to move and get some exercise.

- 6 p.m. to 10 p.m.: kapha time again! Your body cools and you feel a drop in energy as you move toward sleep.
- 10 p.m. to 2 a.m.: Pitta increases, as your body digests food during the night.
- 2 a.m. to 6 a.m.: Vata rises as our bodies prepare to move with the coming of dawn and our awakening.

Based on these cycles, the times of greatest stress for Air types are the hours between two and six, whether during the day or night. In the morning, restless minds awaken vata people early from sleep, while in the afternoon, their energy and mental focus disperse and they become less productive. If you're a vata type, take advantage of this information to plan your days and nights, making the most of your energy's ups and downs.

Besides stress, I think that the biggest reason that Air types become imbalanced is that they ignore the need for rest. Adequate rest is more important for Air types than for others, yet they are least likely to get it because their sleep is easily disrupted and their schedules tend to be erratic. They often average about five to seven hours per night of sleep—but they need more. One of the easiest and quickest ways for vata types to regain their equilibrium is to get a good night's sleep. So if you're a vata who can't sleep, check out the sleep-inducing suggestions in Chapter 6. But more often, Air types *can* sleep, they just don't give themselves enough time to do so.

Here are my recommendations for a daily—and nightly—schedule for Air types:

Twenty-four-hour Schedule for Vata People

- Awaken between 6 a.m. and 7 a.m.
- Take a long, warm shower or bath.
- Allow twenty minutes for conscious breathing or meditation, light stretching, or gentle yoga.
- Eat breakfast between 7 a.m. and 8 a.m.
- Take a fifteen-minute walk after breakfast (and all other meals).
- Work between 8 a.m. or 9 a.m. and 12 noon.
- Take a break midmorning for a walk, stretch, or light snack.
- Eat lunch between noon and 1, preferably in a calm and peaceful environment.

- If possible, take a short nap sometime between 2 p.m. and 4 p.m. At least take a break for twenty to thirty minutes sometime between 3 p.m. and 4 p.m.
- Eat a snack at about 4 p.m.
- Take time to wind down from your day before dinner. This is a good time to get some light exercise.
- Eat dinner by 6 p.m. or 7 p.m., preferably with friends or family— relaxed social time and creating connection are very helpful at balancing vata energies.
- Enjoy a relaxed evening. Go for a walk, read, hang out with friends or family. Evening is also a good time for a spiritual practice, meditation or aromatherapy.
- Go to bed by 10 p.m. or 11 p.m.

⟨₥₥⟩

In addition to a good night's sleep, it is essential that Air types give themselves rest breaks during the day. Follow the section on breaks in Chapter 6 to make sure you know when and how to use break times.

VATA AND THE SEASONS

Just as the day has its cycles, so does the year, with seasons that are more or less conducive to the different energetic types. Vata is aggravated in the fall and winter, when the weather becomes dry, windy, and cold. If you're an Air type, you need to stay warm and keep your skin moist with baths, showers, saunas, and steam rooms, and use moisturizing oils and lotions. This is a particularly important time to follow the dietary suggestions in the chart below, sticking with favored foods and avoiding foods that are not recommended. When the weather is cold and windy, you need to pay particular attention to maintaining your exercise routines and daily schedule.

Your Brain-Healthy Vata Routine: Daily Life for Air Types
- Have a daily routine, even on your days off. When it comes to routine, the problem for Air types is that they often don't have one. Their tendency is to be scattered, rushed, and erratic. Many of my vata patients flounder when they have too much unstructured time, such as when

they are between jobs or after they retire. For most Air types, structure is a good thing, and if they don't have it, their lives tend to become increasingly disarrayed. Think of what happens to air when it isn't contained within an adequate structure. It simply dissipates and disperses. Air within a balloon, or contained and channeled within a bicycle pump, or forced through a radiator can be focused, productive, and effective, a dramatic demonstration of how Air types need schedules, routines, and obligations.

- Don't become too rigid. As we've just seen, Air types need routine. But when their routines are harsh and unforgiving, Vata people tend to get stressed out, and the routine becomes counterproductive, an airless room or a burst balloon. Remember, your goal is balance—structure and rhythm, but not a punishing schedule.

- Make time for rest, renewal, and slowing down. I personally advise Air types to make a regular weekly time to recharge, in the spirit of the ancient suggestion: "Remember the Sabbath, and keep it holy." I'm not suggesting a religious retreat (though that may be a good thing for some) or even an abandonment of all work and routine. But I am advising you to attend to your need to rejuvenate both body and spirit. Take a day each week to go for a walk, see a funny movie, take a luxurious scented bath, or listen to inspiring music. Become more tuned in to the needs of your spirit, and devote at least some time each week to meeting those needs.

- Choose simple, self-nurturing activities, including a slow stroll alone or with a friend; time spent out of doors, especially in the sun; and books and movies that are light, humorous, romantic, entertaining, uplifting, or inspiring. Avoid overly stimulating books and movies during periods of imbalance; no "edge of your seat" thrillers or horror movies.

- Warm baths and showers are great for warming and moistening cool, dry vata, especially when the weather is cold or when you're feeling out of balance.

- Engage your senses with massage—soothing, warming, moistening, and relaxing. Seeing a qualified massage therapist can be a terrific investment, but self-massage works well, too, especially of the neck, shoulders, or feet. Air types should add some sesame oil to their massage oil, try to get massages in the evenings, and stay with gentle, light massage.

- Sound is the second-most-important sense for Air types. Nurture your sense of sound with soothing music such as slow classical, soft jazz, or

New Age. Nature sounds also bring your Air spirits into an almost mag-ical balance—listen to real or recorded babbling brooks, waves crashing upon the shore, birdcalls, or light breezes rustling through the trees.

- Engage your sense of smell, balancing your vata nature with such calm-ing oils as lavender, clary sage, ylang-ylang, geranium, sandalwood, bergamot, and melissa. Ayurveda also recommends basil, clove, and or-ange for vata types.

VATA TYPES:
CHART YOUR PERSONAL JOURNEY

While everyone's life path is unique, certain themes tend to be predom-inant for Air types. Self-acceptance is one prominent issue for such peo-ple, since fear feeds their tendency to feel insecure, unworthy, or ashamed. Believing that they are not good enough as they are draws many vata people to the pursuit of "self-improvement." Ironically, what would *really* be healing and balancing for them is self-acceptance.

Fear likewise drives vatas' frequent belief that they risk not having enough—not enough food, activities, friends, love, or anything else they find valuable. This fear-based belief can lead to a grasping quality, underlying some of the excessive movement and inability to rest that is so unbalancing to Air types. Remembering that *there is enough*—with the help of the techniques in Step Three—can free vatas from this prison of scarcity.

Vatas can likewise benefit from techniques designed to help clear the mind, particularly meditation with awareness of breathing, and then meditation with awareness of thoughts and feelings. The emotions that Air types find particularly "sticky" are fear and insecurity. Learning to release these toxic emotions frees you from their control.

Reflection is also useful for vatas—taking the time to step back, get out of the fray, and reflect on what you are truly thinking and feeling. Using a journal is one way to reflect; finding a therapist or counselor is another. You can also just give yourself some downtime to sit and pon-der a question or even daydream. Just don't move into fretting or worry. That will only undo all the good balancing work you've achieved.

It's not only your mind that needs balancing if you're an Air type. Your spirit also needs sustenance. Inspiration is one key form of nour-ishment for vatas, who thrive on becoming enthusiastic about new things and are drawn into spiritual practices. Inspiration may come from a wide range of sources: friends, books, speakers, tapes, movies, sermons, worship services, prayer. You can also find inspiration within yourself, from listening to your inner voice—a great and never-ending source of inspiration, as we'll see in Chapter 15. Contemplation—time spent in solitude, in relationship with the divine—is also a key balancing practice for vatas. You can experience contemplation through many of the practices described in Step Three as well as through prayer, reflective reading of Scripture, and chanting.

THE BENEFITS OF BALANCE

Although Jeff and I were able to get his Zoloft down to a much smaller dose, he began to notice the lack of serotonin. We boosted his biochemical levels by giving him a twice-daily dose of B-complex vitamins, along with 100 mg of 5-HTP. Jeff's mood rebounded right away. Then we waited until spring to reduce his dosage further, trying to take advantage of the natural rise in mood that occurs for most people in springtime.

Jeff did really well with all the changes he had made, and by springtime, he was able to go off Zoloft entirely. Should he face an especially rocky time in the future, he can always support his mood temporarily with serotonin-boosting supplements or even a low dose of a medication. Meanwhile, though, he'd broken his physiological and psychological dependence on medication.

Jeff's temperament and constitution may make it hard for him to find and maintain balance. After all, it is the very nature of vata, or Air types, to be constantly changing. "Balance" then becomes a moving target. But Jeff found it very helpful to understand and accept his nature, and then to find ways to work with it, learning through observation what threw him off balance so that he could be prepared to cope. As his mind and body calmed down, Jeff also found the time and inner freedom to pursue a more engaged spiritual life, following the mindfulness practices described in Chapter 15. With these, he found more peace than he thought possible, even in the midst of the never-ending stream of stress in which he lived.

Healing for Air Type

Foods:

Overview: regular mealtimes, some protein with each meal, plenty of complex carbohydrates, sweets in moderation.

Recommended Foods:

Dairy: milk and cheese
Meats: turkey, chicken, seafood
Beans and legumes: soy, lentils, chickpeas
Nuts and seeds: walnuts, almonds and almond butter, sesame seeds and tahini, flaxseeds
Grains: whole-grain breads, hot cereals; cooked grains: rice, wheat, or oats
Vegetables: root vegetables: carrots, onions, beets, radishes, turnips, sweet potatoes
Cooked vegetables: asparagus, green beans, okra, garlic
Fruits: sweet, ripe fruits: grapes, melons, oranges, mangoes, berries, cherries, dates, figs, pineapples, plums, nectarines, bananas
Emphasize: warm soups and stews, "comfort foods"

Spices:

anise
basil
cardamom
cinnamon
fennel
ginger
licorice
nutmeg
thyme

Activities:

- seek calm and regularity of schedule
- warmth and moisture
- warm baths, steams, or showers
- drink warm fluids throughout the day
- plenty of sleep, brief naps (if sleeping well at night)
- walks in nature
- seek sunlight
- inspirational or humorous reading
- soft or classical music
- light movies, comedies
- massage
- yoga or qigong
- prayer or meditation

9

SOOTHING FIRE TYPES

Larry, the middle-aged Minnesota farmer whom we met in Chapter 7, was a typical Fire type: energetic and ambitious, someone who cared deeply about the people in his life and the work he did. He originally came to see me because his wife was concerned about his growing irritability and the increasing number of conflicts with his son, while his doctor was disturbed by his consistently high blood pressure, especially given that the men in Larry's family had a history of heart attacks at relatively early ages.

Larry himself knew that something was wrong, but at first he resented the idea that he needed to see a psychiatrist. "I've worked hard all my life, and I'm not about to stop now," he told me, somewhat belligerently. "So if you're here to tell me to take it easy, you can think again."

I could almost see the pitta energy crackling in Larry's tense muscles and flushed skin. When he told me he was suffering from hemorrhoids and high blood pressure, I identified these as further symptoms of a Fire-type imbalance.

"When another person gets stressed," I explained, "he might feel sad, or confused, or slow down. But in that same stressful situation, you tend to speed up, work harder, do more—and become irritable. And your blood pressure, skin, and digestion react accordingly."

PITTA IMBALANCE AND BRAIN CHEMISTRY

Pitta imbalance, in my view, corresponds remarkably well with the Western category of norepinephrine/dopamine excess, or agitated depression. People suffering from this type of depression—probably including Larry—have both a shortage of soothing serotonin and an excess of the stimulating neurotransmitters norepinephrine and dopamine. As a result, they feel anxious, agitated, and on edge—but instead of feeling sad and listless, they feel revved up, overly energized, and pressured.

Fire types can withstand a great deal of stress, but when it's continuous, the body doesn't have the chance to reset itself and recover. In Western biochemical terms, stress causes chemicals known as *catecholamines* to circulate through the bloodstream, along with cortisol and adrenaline, the stimulating stress hormones. Too much stimulation can lead to physical imbalances such as high blood pressure as well as the mental/emotional problems of irritability and becoming overly judgmental. From a Western standpoint, the resulting stressed-out, irritable condition would be diagnosed as depression. It may be difficult for people like this to see themselves as depressed, though their fiery energy translates into anger, irritability, and excessive activity, responses that we don't normally associate with depression. When pitta goes out of balance, Fire types may seem judgmental and critical, compulsive in their routines, and somewhat rigid or controlling. Their bodies respond with elevated blood pressure, flushed skin, and a stomach irritated from too much acid production. It's as though their metabolic fires are literally burning too hot.

When I described a pitta imbalance to Larry, using the fire imagery that Ayurveda suggests, he found himself reluctantly nodding in agreement. "Sometimes," he added, "it's as though there's a fire at my back and I can't stop moving, or it will catch me. But the faster I run to get away from it, the hotter it gets."

⟋☰☰☰⟍

Symptoms of Pitta Imbalance

- feeling angry and irritated
- feeling pressured and overwhelmed with the need to keep working; a "workaholic" pattern of someone who has trouble resting or slowing down
- feeling critical and judgmental of others; a tendency to push others away
- rigid or controlling behavior
- a compulsive tendency to stick to routine and/or to insist that others do so

- trouble falling sleep or staying asleep
- acid indigestion
- flushed or blotchy skin
- hemorrhoids
- diarrhea
- high blood pressure

Factors That Lead to Pitta Imbalance

- stress—particularly ongoing, long-lasting, or intense stress
- pushing too hard at work, or becoming too intensely focused on work
- straining to meet deadlines
- creating unrealistically high expectations for yourself and/or others
- failing to appreciate yourself and/or others
- overeating
- eating too much hot, spicy, greasy, or fermented food
- heat and humidity
- excessive caffeine, nicotine, or other stimulating substances
- insufficient exercise
- failure to identify or express feelings of anger, hostility, or resentment

REBALANCING PITTA ENERGIES

When you think about rebalancing your pitta energies, think of what you'd need to respond to the heat of a fire. Cooling, soothing foods and activities are useful, but so are treatments that help to balance the movement and lightness of a fire. Think of a fire that is raging out of control, consuming everything in its path with its leaping flames, casting flying sparks onto dry grass and withered leaves as they quickly blaze and then crumble into ash. Now think of the same fire brought back into balance, banked within an earthen campfire circle, fed steadily and calmly with heavy logs. As you can see, calmness and substance are just as important as coolness in rebalancing Fire energies.

Fire people can probably handle more stress than Air types, but even they reach a point where the stress gets out of balance. For pitta people, the stressors are often the demands or activities that increase pressure and intensity. So one key rebalancing technique for pitta people—or for other types whose pitta energy is out of balance—is learning to say no. Refusing to take on increased responsibilities and commitments, or learning when you've already taken on too much and need to cut back, can go a long way toward balancing your pitta energy. Ask yourself, "Am I enjoying what I do, or is it a burden?" You know you've taken on too much when you can no longer enjoy activities you once looked forward to—a family outing, a particular task at work, involvement in your local church or synagogue. Watch out for the tendency to let overwork and excessive demands take on a life of their own, or for a heavy schedule to become its own justification. You may accomplish all your tasks with flying colors—but you and your loved ones will pay a price in the anger, irritability, rigidity, or judgmental spirit that you're suddenly bringing to bear on your daily interactions.

Likewise, you can often rebalance pitta energies by reconsidering your expectations of others and resisting the temptation to put undue pressure on them. Pitta energy, like fire, tends to blaze quickly, devouring anything in its path. Sometimes you need that trailblazing fire, and I'm all for drive and ambition when they bring satisfaction, pleasure, and accomplishment. But when they're allowed to run rampant, they can create imbalances in you—and havoc for those around you.

On a more mundane level, when your pitta energies are out of balance, minimize your exposure to heat. Numerous scientific studies have shown a connection between hot, humid weather and explosive violence. There's a reason riots happen more often in the summer than at other seasons of the year and why hot, sweaty athletes have a tendency to lose their tempers.

Finally, pitta imbalance can be eased by cutting back on stimulants like caffeine or nicotine or avoiding them entirely. Why add fuel to a fire? Seek out soothing drinks, like apple, grape, or orange juice, lemonade or limeade, or green tea. Teas featuring the cooling, soothing flavors of cardamom, coriander, licorice, peppermint, and spearmint are also a good choice.

FEEDING YOUR PITTA ENERGIES

One of the contributions of the Ayurvedic perspective is the emphasis on *how* we eat as well as *what* we eat. The best diet in the world can be sabotaged by a stressful or pressured mealtime—and this is particularly true for high-intensity Fire types, who are often tempted to multitask during the meals. In Larry's case, meals had become tension-filled experiences in which he bickered ceaselessly with his son while his wife tried to mediate and his daughter withdrew to stay out of the line of fire.

To support the rebalancing process, I encouraged Larry to eat slowly, without hurry or pressure, in situations where he could enjoy both the food and the company. It was particularly important, I told him, that mealtimes not become the occasions for battles between him and his son. Instead, he should use every family dinner as an occasion to relax and savor the good things in his life. If he had to bring up problems or demands with his son or any other family member, he should save it for after dinner.

As he approached everything in his life, Larry took up these suggestions with discipline, energy, and a strong motivation to succeed. I was happy to hear, when he came back a few weeks later, that meals in his home had become much more pleasant occasions—for both Larry and his family.

Your Brain-Healthy Pitta Diet: How Fire Types Need to Eat

- Eat regularly but moderately. Don't skip meals, and avoid overeating. Fire types have a strong appetite and digestion, but if you eat too much, especially hot and spicy foods, you'll risk imbalance. Think about what causes acid indigestion—pressure, anxiety, spicy foods, and greasy foods. These are all factors that Fire types have to avoid.
- Eat food that is cool or warm, but not overly hot. Your fires are already burning; help them find a comfortable temperature.
- Moderate your consumption of fats and heavy foods. Reduce meat, especially red meat. Generally, you probably need less protein than you think. Remember that imbalanced Fire is more likely to indicate excess than deficiency.
- Favor sweet, bitter, and astringent tastes. See the chart at the end of this chapter for more details.
- Favor cooling, soothing spices: cardamom, coriander, licorice, peppermint, and spearmint.
- Make sure to get at least one daily serving of either lemon or lime. I recommend squeezing one of these fruits into a quart or two of filtered water and drinking it over the course of the day.

- Drink plenty of liquids, especially in summer or when you're engaged in vigorous activity. Favor cold and refreshing drinks. Apple, grape, and orange juice are all good for Fire types. So is tonic water, which tastes a little bitter. Try tonic water and lime in the summer or before meals to cool your fires.
- Eat slowly, without hurry or pressure, enjoying the food. Try not to engage in heated debates during dinner conversation.
- Eat with the seasons. Fire types do well with a summer diet of cool and refreshing foods, high in fresh vegetables and fruits, especially those with high water content like salad greens and melons. You might even continue such a diet throughout the year—but pay particular attention to it in summer, to counter the unbalancing effects of the heat.

Your Brain-Healthy Pitta Detox: How Fire Types Need to Cleanse
- Follow the detox suggestions I shared in Chapter 6, with a special focus on saunas and steam baths. If you're feeling out of balance, you might aim for a twenty-minute sauna once or twice a week.

FANNING THE FLAMES: EXERCISE FOR FIRE TYPES

Fire types tend to be fairly athletic and need to exercise in order to feel good. Certainly Larry had always benefited from the vigorous work he'd done on his farm. When he came to me, however, it was midwinter, and although he'd been working extremely hard, he hadn't been getting the kind of workout he needed. As a result, the stress and tension had built up to a dangerous degree, expressing itself physically in high blood pressure and muscle pain and emotionally in Larry's anger and irritability.

I recommended that Larry find a sport or activity he liked and engage in it at least four or five times a week. I warned him, though, that he should choose a moderate-intensity exercise, preferably one that didn't involve too much competition. Overdoing it by pushing too hard or getting caught up in heated competition are the typical downfalls of Fire types.

Larry got into the habit of taking a brisk walk during the winter and a light jog in the summer. I suggested that he consider swimming—especially good for Fire types because the body stays fairly cool—as well as winter sports like skiing or skating. I also encouraged him to consider rowing, canoeing, tennis, or golf, though I warned him to avoid playing with particularly competitive partners. Although none of these exercise suggestions quite "caught fire" with Larry, he promised to consider them if walking and jogging didn't offer him sufficient relief from stress.

Your Brain-Healthy Pitta Exercise Plan: Activities for Fire Types
- Notice whether or not you're enjoying the exercise or sport you've chosen. If not, slow down, switch gears, and see if you can drop the intensity level a bit. Or find another activity that you enjoy more.
- Fire types tend to like sports because of the skill level required and the competition involved. But be careful not to allow your drive and competitiveness to take control. Intense competition creates a fire imbalance. Have you ever seen an athlete start cursing or throwing down a tennis racket or golf club? That's when the competitive fires are burning too brightly, eating away at the Fire types. Find a way of moving your body that involves only your own pleasure, not the attempt to reach a predetermined goal.
- Favor a repetitive activity, such as a moderate walk, a light run, or a swim, which has the added advantage of cooling the body. Fire types also do well with winter sports, including all forms of skiing or skating.

BREATHING AND BIORHYTHMS FOR FIRE TYPES

Fire types run the risk of getting overly regimented and perhaps rigid about their schedule and routine, letting their routine run them instead of feeling in charge of their schedule and activities. They need to remember to take down time, to give themselves time away from their work.

Like many Fire types, Larry had the tendency to become a workaholic, one of the classic Type A personalities who are so driven and ambitious that they seem to lose the ability to slow down at all. In Larry's case, it seemed there was always something to do—bills to pay, equipment to order, catalogs to peruse, markets to research. I urged Larry to avoid working in the evening and on weekends. Like most Fire types, he found this hard advice to follow—but he agreed to try my plan for two weeks. When we spoke later, he was torn.

"I really enjoyed myself much more than I thought I would," he admitted. "And my wife was real happy that I was around more. But I feel like I'm not getting enough done."

I suggested that Larry give the "no-after-hours" policy another two or three weeks. If after that time he wanted to start adding in extra activities, he could try working one evening a week or part of a weekend day. The goal, I told him, was to make sure he was actually choosing to work, in response to either a pressing need or the pleasure it gave him. The danger was that he'd end up feeling that he "needed to work" all the time, simply because the routine took on a life of its own. His motto, I suggested, should be the ancient truism "All things in moderation."

Balancing Your Fire Energy Through Breathing

Like vata types, pitta people can benefit a great deal from the Calming Breath Technique described in Chapter 6. To balance your pitta energy, you might also try left nostril breathing. Inhale through your left nostril, and exhale through the right. Use your thumb and forefinger to gently close the appropriate nostril. The practice seems to have a calming effect on imbalanced pitta energy.

CIRCADIAN RHYTHMS AND PITTA ENERGY

In the previous chapter, I described the Ayurvedic understanding of the day's circadian rhythms. As you can see on pages 142 `and 143, the time periods from ten to two in both mornings and evenings, are when Fire types can become most easily stressed. During midday, they may be more likely to "fly off the handle," feeling stressed, short-tempered, or overwhelmed. At night, they may have trouble sleeping during those hours if they feel pressured by the day's activities. In that case, Fire types should adopt a good bedtime routine, because they tend to sleep more than Air types, getting perhaps six to eight hours of sleep per night.

Here's how I think Fire types can best organize their daily cycle:

෧ᢍᢍᢍᢂ

Twenty-four-hour Schedule for Pitta People

- Awaken between 6 a.m. and 7 a.m.
- Take a cool shower or bath.
- Devote twenty minutes to conscious breathing or meditation, exercise, or yoga. Early morning can be a good time for pittas to engage in vigorous exercise because it is the coolest time of day.
- Eat breakfast between 7 a.m. and 8 a.m.
- Take a fifteen-minute walk after breakfast—and every meal.
- Perform your most intense, demanding, or frustrating work between 8 a.m. and 10 a.m.
- Take a midmorning break for a walk, some stretching, or a light snack.
- Try to perform less stressful, more creative work between 10 a.m. and noon.
- Eat lunch between noon and 1 p.m., preferably in a calm and peaceful environment. Midday is also a good time for exercise if it is not too hot.
- Take a twenty- to thirty-minute break sometime between 3 p.m. and 4 p.m. Have a light, refreshing snack at about 3 p.m.
- As the afternoon winds down, take time to review your day, assessing what went well and planning for the next day. If you do this before you leave work, you'll find it easier to leave work behind.
- Wind down from the day before dinner. Light exercise is okay at this time of day, but don't do anything too strenuous or competitive.
- Eat dinner by 6 p.m. or 7 p.m., preferably with friends or family. The warm, social connections you have with loved ones are very helpful for balancing pitta energy.
- Enjoy a relaxed evening. Go for a walk, read, hang out with friends or family. Evening is a good time for a spiritual practice, meditation, or aromatherapy. Fire types will also benefit enormously from doing some yoga during this time.
- Go to bed by 10 p.m. or 11 p.m. If you need to establish a bedtime routine to help you sleep, a cooling bath is useful for Fire types.

෧ᢍᢍᢍᢂ

PITTA AND THE SEASONS

Fire types often feel more easily aggravated in the summer, when the hot, dry weather tends to inflame their tempers and irritate their spirits. If you're a pitta person, take it easy in the summer. Try to slow down and spend plenty of time just relaxing with family and friends. Hours spent in a pool or by a lake are hours well spent.

I encourage most Fire types to choose the cool of the day for more vigorous activities like sports or exercise. Larry pointed out that summer was a busy time on his farm, and he didn't have the option of waiting until the weather cooled to tend to his fields and livestock. I suggested that he make sure to refresh himself with plenty of filtered water or tonic water and lemon or lime, and that he find cool places for eating lunch and snacks throughout the day.

Your Brain-Healthy Pitta Routine: Daily Life for Fire Types
- What works best for pitta types is flexibility in routine, with plenty of built-in downtime. Pitta people also need to make sure they've scheduled activities or periods when their focus is on being thoughtful and attentive to others, to get them out of a focus on themselves.
- Refreshing breaks for pitta types include taking a cool shower or bath, eating a light snack of yogurt or fresh fruit, and drinking some cool water or juice.
- Walks are wonderful recreation for pitta people, either alone or with a friend. Get outside and enjoy nature, but avoid prolonged periods in the sun. And try to make your focus on pleasure, not on achieving a goal. Instead of walking briskly to reach a distant destination, let yourself just stroll and enjoy the view.
- Laugh a lot. For you Fire types, or for other types whose pitta energies are out of balance, laughter truly is the best medicine. Seek out sources of humor, such as comics, humorous books, funny friends, or comedians.
- Look for books or movies that are funny, romantic, or dramatic. Avoid those that are overstimulating, violent, or disturbing.
- Engage your senses, particularly sight, which is the most engaged sense for Fire types. Enjoy great art or the beauty of nature. It is very soothing for Fire types to view a lovely sunset, look out over an impressive vista, or simply to contemplate the beauty of a single flower. Visual arts, like drawing, painting, or photography are good choices for Fire hobbies.

- Massage can be terrifically healing for Fire people. Use sunflower oil to cool your fiery energies and try to schedule your sessions in the afternoon, after your "high-stress" time of 2 p.m. has passed. Use a light technique. Vigorous or invasive deep-tissue massage can inflame rather than sooth pitta energies.

- Aromatherapy techniques can also be helpful to pitta people, particularly the cooling oils mint, jasmine, and sandalwood.

- Mind-body exercises are great to help Fire types unwind. Yoga is especially good because it allows pitta people to expend some of their energy and meet some of their needs for athletic challenge while building flexibility and agility to counteract the Fire type's tendency to rigidity. Choose a teacher and type of yoga that is peaceful and not overly driven, and don't get too focused on achievement or competing with others in the class.

- When approached with moderate intensity, tai chi can also be a great fit for Fire types. The movements are flowing and give the whole body a light workout without heating it up too much. Again, look for a teacher who has a laid-back approach to it so that the practice remains a pleasurable pursuit rather than another arena of intense competition.

- Aikido is a somewhat less well-known martial art that originated in Japan. It involves a fairly intense workout but can be great for Fire types because of its emphasis on the peaceful resolution of conflict. The aikido philosophy embraces the cultivation of inner peace and nonviolence, and the movements teach the practitioners to flow with the energy of the attacker. The right aikido instructor can teach Fire types to reduce their own anger, to pay more attention to the other, to give ground or "lose" gracefully, and even to "win" through loss.

PITTA TYPES:
EXPLORING YOUR PERSONAL JOURNEY

One of the key themes for many Fire types is *acceptance of others*. I often feel that the difficulty many Fire types have with this concept is rooted in their fear that they won't achieve their own ambitions. When this fear gets out of control, the Fire rages and the pitta person can become self-centered, even aggressive. In fact, Fire types can become so intensely driven and self-focused that they scarcely notice that others exist. Ironically, they may be the happiest of all when they manage to rebalance their energies by taking the focus off themselves and remembering that there are others who also matter.

Thus, the cultivation of compassion, which is a work of the heart, provides the perfect antidote to cool the fires of ambition. Compassion moves you out of yourself and into the life of another to such a degree that the only possible response is love. Fire types may find it particularly helpful to try some of the techniques from Step Three: meditation, reflection, generosity toward others, and the heart-opening exercise I describe in Chapter 15. Because Fire types thrive on all things visual, adding a visual element to your meditation or spiritual practice can be both grounding and inspiring. You might want to create a personal altar space with pictures of loved ones or of important spiritual figures, pieces of art, and objects from nature. You can use a candle or a sacred object to focus on during your time for prayer or meditation. Or, with your eyes closed, visualize being in a particular setting, with a certain person, or undergoing some sort of desirable experience.

ACHIEVING PITTA BALANCE

When Larry began to apply a wide range of pitta-balancing suggestions, he found that almost immediately he felt calmer and more relaxed. Although his problems hadn't gone away, he felt as though he'd expanded into a larger space, where there was more room and time to deal with them. The pressure—so common to pitta types—had lifted, and in his new, cooler mode, he felt better equipped to find solutions.

Fire types tend to be so driven that their greatest tendency is to do too much. By doing too much, they fill the space that surrounds their lives and can easily begin to feel confined. Like Larry, they often get so caught up in the intensity of what they're doing that they fail to honor the natural rhythms of activity followed by inactivity. So it became important for Larry to remember that, while he could still work hard, he had to stop all the *doing* once in a while and give himself a chance to simply *be*. After a lifetime of striving, slowing down was a challenge for Larry. But he realized that this was the only way he could choose to open up spaces in his life for something other than work and then create the life he wanted from this point forward.

Healing for Fire Type

Foods:
Overview: less protein, lighter foods with high water content

Recommended Foods:
Dairy: milk, egg whites
Meats: smaller servings of chicken, turkey, shrimp
Beans and legumes: tofu
Nuts and seeds: pumpkin and sunflower seeds
Grains: barley, oats, wheat, white rice
Vegetables: green, leafy vegetables and salads
Fruits: apples, cherries, grapes, mangoes, melons, oranges, pears, pineapple, plums, raisins

Spices:
cardamom
coriander (cilantro)
cinnamon
cumin
dill
fennel
lemon and lime
peppermint
saffron
spearmint
turmeric

Activities:
- seek moderation and balance of activity with rest
- shorter, cooler showers and baths
- drink cool beverages, plenty of water
- eat smaller amounts more often
- plenty of time in nature (though avoid midday heat)
- moderate but regular exercise for twenty to thirty minutes at a time
- get plenty of laughter and humor
- meditation
- tai chi or yoga

10
MOVING EARTH TYPES

Cindy, as you recall, was a fifty-year-old woman who had spent a lifetime struggling with both weight and depression. She had benefited from a number of the diet, exercise, and lifestyle changes that I've described in Step One. But it was the Ayurvedic Mind-Body approach that really inspired her.

According to Ayurveda, Cindy was a classic Earth type, a true kapha—heavy, sturdy, and stable, whose chief strength and most frustrating weakness was the difficulty of getting her to move. When Cindy was at her best, her kapha energies made her loving, nurturing, strong, and reliable—a true earth mother. When she struggled with kapha imbalances, however, she was depressed, weighed down with extra flesh, sluggish, and slow-moving, as though she were slogging through mud or carrying the world on her shoulders.

Cindy liked the earth-inspired images of Ayurveda more than the medical terminology or the psychological language that she'd encountered from her previous physicians and psychiatrists. "I feel that we're talking about all of me," she told me once. "I'm not just this problem or that problem—I'm a whole package."

KAPHA IMBALANCE AND BRAIN CHEMISTRY

In Western terms, kapha imbalance bears a remarkable resemblance to depression caused by a norepinephrine/dopamine deficiency. Both have similar symptoms: depressed mood, low energy, a tendency to sleep more, weight gain, withdrawal, a kind of passivity, decreased sex drive, impotence or frigidity, slowed thoughts, poor memory, and sometimes even suicidal feelings. As we saw in Chapter 2, there are clear biochemical causes for these symptoms. But I like the Ayurvedic explanation as well.

According to Ayurveda, kapha people become imbalanced when they have too little energy to keep moving. When out of balance, they tend to feel sluggish and lethargic. They sleep too much and have difficulty waking. They often gain weight and may even become obese. And on a psychological level, they can become stubborn, set in their ways, dependent, and clingy.

When a kapha imbalance continues too long, it becomes depression, a condition marked by a lack of energy and motivation, the tendency to withdraw and to lose interest in the world, difficulty concentrating, and trouble remaining focused and alert. I sometimes think of depressed kapha types as literally sinking into the earth, with too little energy or motivation to pull themselves out of the damp ground in which they are mired. In fact, kapha energies—whether healthy or depressed—are marked by moisture, coolness, and heaviness, and they are almost always slow to move. So when kapha goes out of balance, we seek treatments to add dryness, warmth, lightness, and stimulating energy.

⟨⟩

Symptoms of Kapha Imbalance

- feeling sluggish and listless
- fatigue
- feeling unmotivated and pessimistic, a kind of "what's the use?" attitude
- slow-moving or unfocused behavior
- difficulty concentrating
- memory problems
- a compulsive tendency to stick to routine and be unable to imagine a way out
- dependency on familiar people, places, and situations
- excessive sleeping and/or trouble waking up in the mornings
- weight gain and tendency toward obesity
- passivity
- decreased sex drive and/or impotence/frigidity

⟨⟩

Kapha is the most stable of the three types. But when kapha types do lose their equilibrium, they have the most difficulty regaining it. As Cindy and I agreed, her greatest strengths were also her greatest weaknesses. The very stability and solidity that made her such a nurturing parent and reliable worker were now making it difficult for her to lose weight, regain her energy, and make the needed changes in her life that would free her from her depression.

Because kapha imbalances take so long to develop, it can be difficult to see them clearly. Here are some of the factors that often create kapha imbalance:

⁂

Factors That Lead to Kapha Imbalance

- prolonged or severe stress; Earth types can withstand more stress than their Fire or Air counterparts, but if stress lasts long enough or is intense enough, they'll eventually lose their balance.
- prolonged lack of pressure, or understimulation, as in a dull job or a lifeless marriage
- relationships marked by excessive dependency or clinging
- withdrawing, not wanting to call people or to leave home, having too little contact with others
- taking sedating or depressant chemicals, such as alcohol, sleeping pills, and even many antidepressants, especially at higher doses
- lack of movement, too little exercise
- excess sleep, especially sleeping in late in the morning
- eating too much and becoming overweight
- eating too many sweet, salty, or fatty foods, or indulging in excess dairy products
- cold and damp weather, as in winter and spring; SAD is often a kapha imbalance

⁂

REBALANCING KAPHA ENERGIES

I always suggest to my patients that they begin with the simplest solutions. So if you're a kapha type or a kapha combination and you're feeling stuck, start by getting rid of anything that might tend to sedate you: alcohol, marijuana, antihistamines and similar over-the-counter medications, St. John's wort, kava and other herbs, and even some of the antidepressant medications. *Of course you must never—I repeat, never—stop taking prescription antidepressants or even reduce your dosage without first consulting your doctor.* But if you are taking antidepressants and your depression seems to be getting worse, ask your doctor about whether your dosage can be reduced, particularly if you're feeling slow, listless, or sedated.

Sleep can seem very attractive to Earth people, but too much sleep is a common cause of imbalance. People with excess kapha are often amazed to find out how much more alert and energetic they can feel just by cutting back on sleep for a few days. See the suggestions I made for hypersomnia in Chapter 6, or try some of these recommendations:

⟨꩜⟩

Steps to Reduce Excessive Sleep

1. Make sure to get up at the same time every day, preferably between 6 a.m. and 8 a.m. If you let yourself sleep later, you'll get out of alignment with the earth's rhythm and feel more sluggish. This can occur even with one day of "sleeping in," so try to avoid that even on weekends.

2. Set your alarm fifteen minutes earlier each day until you get to your chosen wake-up time. If an alarm doesn't wake you, set another across the room so that you have to get up to shut it off.

3. If you still have trouble waking, try a dawn simulator at your bedside. The gradually brightening light sends a strong signal to the brain to awaken. It is also very helpful to use bright light (a SAD light) for twenty to thirty minutes just after arising.

4. Once you can get up at a consistent hour, you will likely be sleeping between seven to nine hours each night. But if you're still getting more than nine hours of sleep because you fall asleep too early, try to stay awake fifteen minutes later each night. It may help to use bright light exposure late in the day, between 5 p.m. and 7 p.m., to push back the time that you fall asleep.

5. Avoid naps until your nighttime sleep is regulated at a consistent seven to nine hours per night. If you must nap, limit your siestas to

thirty minutes or less, or you will again notice that you feel more sluggish.

∽⟨⟩∼

Meanwhile, take a long, hard look at your daily routine. Have you fallen into a rut? Do something different: Eat lunch in a new restaurant, walk to work instead of taking the bus, go off on a Saturday afternoon to someplace you've never been before. Or if you need to make bigger changes, talk to your boss, your spouse, your family to shift a pattern that's no longer working for you.

Be sure, too, that you're not clinging to relationships that aren't serving you well, or becoming overly dependent on the people you love. Kapha types are talented at relationships, establishing long-lasting ties with loved ones, family members, and friends. But sometimes Earth types must learn to let go, or to demand significant changes within a relationship.

Cindy realized that she had gotten into a rut with her husband. Although early in their marriage they'd both enjoyed a certain amount of separate socializing, Cindy discovered that somehow, she almost never saw her husband. An active Fire type, he always seemed to be busy with work, church activities, or a project with one of the kids. But she had grown so used to the situation that she barely was aware that it bothered her. Only later, after engaging in the mindfulness work I describe in Step Three, did Cindy begin to understand how angry, sad, and frustrated she was by many aspects of her marriage. She had told herself that "it didn't matter"—and her kapha imbalance was the result.

FEEDING YOUR KAPHA ENERGIES

I introduced Cindy to the Ayurvedic theory of the six types of flavor—sweet, sour, salty, bitter, pungent, and astringent. I encouraged her to favor kapha-pacifying foods, those with bitter, pungent, and astringent flavors. I explained that she would find it stimulating to pique her taste buds with bitter leafy greens—kale, arugula, escarole, and the like; the pungent flavors of onion, ginger, garlic, and cayenne; and the astringent vegetables broccoli, cauliflower, cabbage, and brussels sprouts.

Cindy found that her altered diet did seem to wake up her taste buds while restoring some of her vigor. She realized that the sweet, salty foods she cherished were indeed soothing—but now she needed less to be calmed and comforted than to be inspired and energized. She also found that just the effort involved in making these dietary changes "woke her up"—that creating new habits of shopping, cooking, and eating were helping her get out of her rut.

Your Brain-Healthy Kapha Diet: How Earth Types Need to Eat

- Eat less. If you're an Earth type, you tend to put on weight, and both your body and your energies are weighed down accordingly. Think about taking in fewer calories and switching from heavier to lighter foods, particularly when you are feeling depressed, sluggish, or out of tune with the world around you.
- Reduce or avoid sweets. Many of my kapha patients have told me that they seem to gain weight easily even when they don't eat much. They may be getting too many sweets and starchy foods, consuming processed sugar and refined carbohydrates. Earth types seem poorly equipped to handle these substances, which their body easily stores as fat.
- Generally, you should consume more protein and less carbohydrates than the other two types. Check out Chapter 4 and follow the diet for norepi/dopa deficiency.
- Earth types have a generally slower metabolism and can go longer than the other types between meals without feeling imbalanced. This is the only type that can get away with skipping breakfast, though I still don't recommend it. I do recommend a low-calorie, high-protein breakfast, such as a protein/fruit/juice shake or a couple of hard-boiled eggs and a dish of berries. Generally, choose fruits and juices that aren't overly sweet, and of course stay well away from sweetened fruit juice, which can set off blood-sugar imbalances and create a craving for sugar.
- Go for lots of variety in your diet. Remember, in pretty much every area of life, Earth types have to be careful about not getting into a rut. Remind yourself that variety is literally the spice of life by including in your diet a wide range of tastes, textures, food groups—and spices.
- Cut back on sweet, salty, and sour foods, including ice cream, most desserts, chips, white breads, pastas, and all dairy products except unsweetened yogurt, kefir (a kind of liquid yogurt), and low-fat cottage cheese. Skim milk in moderation is okay, but you should still aim for less dairy, overall. Instead, favor pungent, bitter, and astringent foods, which still stimulate you and help you regain your lost energy. (See the

table below for more detail on how to incorporate these flavors into your diet.)

- Eat slowly and mindfully. Besides helping you digest your food, this will also help you realize when you've had enough. You'll be less likely to overeat—and more likely to increase the pleasure you take in the sensual aspects of food, including taste, texture, and aroma.
- Favor warm drinks and avoid putting ice in your drinks, including water. Ginger tea will stimulate your taste buds while aiding in digestion. Green tea can stimulate your system and provide you with lots of antioxidants. Even black tea can perk you up and keep your energy moving.

Your Brain-Healthy Kapha Detox: How Earth Types Need to Cleanse

Follow the detox suggestions I shared in Chapter 6, with these special suggestions for kapha types:

- Because of their constitution, Earth types may undertake a longer fast than the other types, going without food for up to a week. However, I would recommend undertaking any fast of more than two days under appropriate supervision *only*. For either shorter or longer juice fasts, apple and cranberry are good choices.
- Dry saunas are particularly useful for Earth types. You can take one any time of year, but you'll appreciate them most from winter through early spring, when they can help you lose some of the kapha moisture that weighs on your body and spirit. I also recommend saunas during your detox month: at least a few times per week, or up to twenty to thirty minutes once or twice a day if you've got easy access to a sauna.

EXERCISING YOUR KAPHA NATURE

Earth types can be strong and athletic, especially when young. But their tendency to become sedentary and gain weight as adults makes exercise of utmost importance for staying in balance.

Earth types also have the most to gain from regular exercise. For them, exercise should be vigorous, requiring them to push themselves and go a bit beyond their "comfort zone." Of course they should make sure to take precautions to avoid injury, although they are the most durable of the three types and the least likely to get injured. However, since they've often gotten out of shape by avoiding exercise, they must be particularly careful when resuming an exercise routine, and should check with their physicians if there is any concern about the health of their hearts.

As we saw in Chapter 6, exercise was a major key to Cindy's renewed health and vigor. Engaging in exercise that required Cindy to break a sweat, to push herself, and to move quickly really helped wake up her kapha energies, even as it replenished her depleted stores of norepinephrine and dopamine. Both kapha types and people suffering from unbalanced kapha energies should follow my suggestions in Chapter 6 for the exercise suited to restore norepi/dopa depletion.

Your Brain-Healthy Kapha Exercise Plan: Activities for Earth Types

- Try to move and break a sweat almost every day. If you have the time and are so inclined, you can benefit by spending more time in exercise than the other types—from forty-five to sixty minutes a day.
- Do both aerobic and weight training. Aerobic classes with vigorous movements and stimulating music can work great for Earth types. Weight training can strengthen and tone your muscles, helping you carry any extra weight more easily while trimming and refining your bodies. Weight training will help you both to feel better physically and to feel better about yourself.
- Participating in competitive sports can also be helpful for kapha people. Such activity tends to be more stimulating and gets the energy flowing.
- Exciting outdoor activities, even those with a mild element of risk, can help energize Earth types. Examples might include rock climbing, white-water rafting, sea kayaking, mountain biking. Anyone for parachuting?

BREATHING AND BIORHYTHMS FOR EARTH TYPES

Like most kapha types who are struggling with depression, Cindy benefited from establishing a daily routine emphasizing regularity, less sleep, and an earlier rising time. Figuring out how much regularity Cindy needed required a delicate balancing act, to be sure. Earth types run into problems when routine becomes, too, well, *routine*. When their days are too much the same, one after another, their energy stagnates and life seems dull. They could use a little of the spontaneity of the Air types or the drive of the Fire types. But Earth types can also let lack of structure lead them into lethargy and sluggishness. Too little movement, with or without structure, is the common pitfall of this constitution. Their motto should be "A rolling stone gathers no moss."

Cindy used the Energizing Breath Technique described in Chapter 6 to give herself a boost each morning and early afternoon, right after her session with the light box, which she used to combat SAD. She also relied on this useful technique whenever she felt depressed or sluggish or when she had difficulty concentrating.

Balancing Your Earth Energy Through Breathing

In addition to the Energizing Breath Technique, Earth types can benefit from right nostril breathing. Inhale through the right nostril, and exhale through the left, covering whichever nostril you're not using with your thumb and forefinger. Ayurvedic practitioners and yogis believe that the right nostril focus helps balance kapha energy.

CIRCADIAN RHYTHMS AND KAPHA ENERGY

In Chapter 8, I described the Ayurvedic understanding of the day's circadian rhythms. As you can see on pages 142 to 143, the times of greatest stress for Earth types are the hours between six and ten. In the morning, Earth types tend to be sluggish until 10 a.m., with difficulty getting out of bed and beginning their day. In the evening, their energy and mental focus begin to diminish between six and ten as they prepare to sleep. Some people with kapha imbalance become very sleepy in the evening, especially in the winter months. Regardless of season, it is normal for Earth types to get more sleep than the others, averaging perhaps eight to nine hours a day. But if they sleep longer than that, the fog of heaviness quickly drifts in.

Here's how Earth types might best arrange their days and nights:

⊙⫘⊙

Twenty-four-hour Schedule for Kapha People

- Awaken between 6 a.m. and 8 a.m. If morning sluggishness is a problem, get up by 6 a.m. so you're already awake when the kapha period begins.
- Take a warm shower.
- Spend thirty minutes on energizing breathing or meditation, or on some fairly vigorous exercise like yoga or running. In winter, this would be a good time for bright light exposure.
- Eat a light breakfast between 7 a.m. and 9 a.m.
- Take a short walk of about fifteen minutes after each meal.
- Work from 9 a.m. to noon, but include a midmorning break for a walk, stretch, or light snack.
- Eat lunch between noon and one, preferably in a warm and energizing environment. Lunch should be your heaviest meal of the day, so you have many hours to burn off the food before going to sleep. The noon hour might also be a good time for a vigorous walk or another form of exercise.
- Avoid napping. Extra sleep aggravates kapha and may exacerbate fatigue and weight gain.
- Work from 1 p.m. to 5 p.m. But break up your afternoon with some tea and perhaps have a high-protein snack at about 4 p.m.
- Take time to wind down from the day before dinner. This is a good time to get some more exercise.
- Eat dinner by 6 p.m. or 7 p.m., preferably with friends or family. Keep this meal light.
- Enjoy a stimulating evening. Join groups, take a class (possibly yoga or aerobics), see a good movie, or go out to hear some music. Try to seek out activities, especially in winter months. Avoid the temptation to sit at home watching TV and snacking. Minimize evening eating.
- Late evening is a good time for a spiritual practice, meditation, or aromatherapy.
- Go to bed by 10 p.m. or 11 p.m.

⊙⫘⊙

KAPHA AND THE SEASONS

As Cindy had discovered, kapha is aggravated in winter, when the world seems cold and dark. Early spring—cool and damp—can also aggravate Earth types, as can any cool, damp weather.

Cindy also struggled with SAD, as we have seen, a typical Earth type imbalance to winter's lack of sunlight. She quickly learned that as soon as she noticed herself slowing down, feeling sluggish, gaining weight, and wanting to sleep too much, it was time to pull out the light box and take the other measures referred to in Chapter 6. Happily, she, like many kapha types, was eventually able to overcome her tendency to SAD through these techniques plus diet, breathing, and the other Earth-balancing suggestions described in this chapter.

Your Brain-Healthy Kapha Routine: Daily Life for Earth Types
- What works best for Earth types is variety within routine. Earth types should also make a point of finding people and activities that interest and stimulate them. Just as the clogged and muddy stream needs fresh water to keep the energy flowing, so do kapha people need friends, teachers, colleagues, and activities to inspire them to keep moving.

Quick Energizers for Kapha Types
- Try a few minutes of the Energizing Breath Technique or some right nostril breathing.
- Eat a small high-protein snack or some spicy food.
- Drink something warm: water with lemon and a little honey, an herbal tea (try ginger, ginseng, or African red bush), or green tea.
- Do a few quick calisthenics—anything to warm up the body and move some energy through it.

- Simple pleasures for Earth types include a brisk walk alone or, better yet, with a walking partner. Get outside and enjoy nature, particularly if you can seek warmth and the sun.
- A new hobby, class, or adventure—any type of new activity—can shake

things up for Earth types. Dance and music, with their movement and
endless variety, make excellent lifelong pursuits.

- Look for books and movies that are dramatic, thrilling, or action-
packed. Especially when you're depressed, avoid slow-moving, sad, and
sentimental stories.

- Taste and smell are the senses that most engage Earth types. Perhaps
that is one of the reasons why they find it hard to avoid weight gain—
they get trapped into getting most of their stimulation from taste. Instead of quantity, go for more interesting foods. Try a new type of
cuisine or order an unfamiliar food, especially something spicy or hot.
Try to get more of your stimulation from food's aroma and focus on
mindful eating for enhanced pleasure without all the calories.

- Massage can be helpful for Earth types, who benefit most from morning
rubdowns. They can tolerate a deep, invigorating type of massage, ideally with corn or calamus-root oil, or even a dry massage without oil.

- Aromatherapy can also lift the spirits and boost the energy of kapha
people. Oils that improve mood include basil, cinnamon, coriander,
patchouli, peppermint, rose, jasmine, neroli, melissa, ylang-ylang, sandalwood, thyme, citrus oils (grapefruit, lime, mandarin, bergamot),
geranium, and lavender. Eucalyptus both boosts mood and helps clear
sinus congestion, a common complaint of Earth types.

- Mind-body integrative exercises most helpful for Earth types might include yoga, to help generate and move energy, qigong, and such martial
arts as karate, tae kwon do, aikido, and kickboxing. Look for more vigorous forms of yoga, such as those done in a heated room (Bikram yoga
is one such type). Likewise, qigong helps generate energy and keep it
flowing, which may help mobilize an Earth type. Martial arts may suit
Earth types because of the physical challenge and stimulating nature of
the practice. Earth types are already well grounded, which gives them
an immediate martial-arts advantage, and further study can help them
learn to mobilize their bodies and use their energy. The competition
found in some forms of martial art can also be appropriately energizing
for Earth types.

- High-speed activities are also quite stimulating. Consider righting your
kapha imbalance with boating, motorcycling, skydiving, bungee jumping, or a ride on a roller coaster.

- Music can stimulate energies as well, especially rock and roll, or pas-
sionate classical pieces.

Note: Many depressed people become intolerant of *any* arousal, even though ultimately, arousal is what they need. In response to their difficulties, however, they isolate themselves and restrict their activities. If you feel anxious or irritable at the very thought of the kinds of stimulating activities I've described, start slowly, adding stimulation in small doses. Otherwise, you may feel overloaded and withdraw further.

KAPHA TYPES:
EXPLORING YOUR PERSONAL JOURNEY

Issues that tend to be significant for Earth types include struggling to accept what is. Earth types seem unusually prone to getting caught in the darkness of what the Buddhists call delusion—the inability or unwillingness to see things as they really are. This can lead to a "head-in-the-sand" mentality in which a kapha person allows problems to continue, either because they seem to have always been present or because the kapha person is unwilling to accept that they really *are* problems. The way out is to embrace and cultivate mindfulness, the ability to be fully in each moment with clear seeing and accepting of what is. (You can read more about these issues in Step Three.)

Earth types also have the tendency to accumulate, to store more than is needed. They often hold on to extra weight, discredited ideas, unhealthy relationships, dissatisfying jobs, or problematic personal situations. The way out may be to let go of the unnecessary, to practice detachment, and to unclutter the mind as well as the environment. Meditation, reflection, and letting go can all be enormously helpful for Earth types, who can find it especially useful to return frequently to the basic spiritual question "What is life-giving and what is death-dealing or lifeless at this moment in my life?"

RESTORING KAPHA BALANCE

Cindy benefited enormously from the kapha balancing techniques I've described. The physical interventions—diet, supplements, exercise, and using the light box—boosted her energy and her mood, opening her to new possibilities in her life and to new approaches to self-care. They were the gateway to the spiritual and emotional balancing she undertook, particularly the mindfulness work I'll describe in subsequent chapters. With its combination of treatments geared to mind, body, and spirit, the Ayurvedic approach enabled Cindy to address her problems on many fronts—with slow but steady success.

Healing for Earth Type

Foods:
Overview: more protein, fewer carbohydrates, very few sweets or fats

Recommended Foods:
Dairy: skim milk
Meats: low-fat meats
Beans and legumes: all are fine
Nuts and Seeds: sunflower and pumpkin seeds
Grains: barley, buckwheat, corn, millet, rye
Vegetables: all are okay, many may be eaten raw. Eat fewer of those with high glycemic index (e.g., potatoes and sweet potatoes).
Fruits: apples, pears, apricots, cranberries

Spices:
basil
black or cayenne pepper
cardamom
celery seeds
cinnamon
cloves
ginger
lemon
mustard
parsley
peppermint
sage
spearmint
thyme

Activities:
- seek stimulation and variety
- light meals
- regular, vigorous, or competitive exercise
- travel, meeting new people, trying new things
- dry heat (e.g., sauna)
- drink moderate amounts of warm fluids (may use some caffeine)
- outdoor adventures: boating, climbing, rafting, skiing
- action movies, mysteries
- lively music, dancing
- consider a martial art or vigorous form of yoga

STEP THREE:

Discover Your Buddhist
Emotional Type

11

BUDDHIST WISDOM: WHICH TYPE ARE YOU?

So far, we've focused on the physical: the Western brain-chemistry focus and the Ayurvedic tradition of Mind-Body medicine that can help you identify the food, supplements, exercise, and habits to help you overcome your depression.

Now, without forgetting the importance of this groundedness in the body, we're going to move into more psychological and spiritual realms. But before we begin, I want to clear up two common misconceptions that I often encounter.

First, I am not trying to convert you to Buddhism or to any type of religious practice. Both my own and my patients' interest in this approach comes from the broadest possible perspective, that of desiring to see the world clearly and to understand our own relationship to it. So whether you follow a Buddhist tradition, a different spiritual practice, or no spiritual practice at all, you can still join me in a study of Buddhist psychology and the mindfulness techniques it has inspired.

Second, although we're now moving into psychological and emotional realms, I don't want you to forget the importance of your body. Food, exercise, sleep, and biorhythms are all enormously important components of our lives, and I've seen my patients make remarkable progress when we worked within those realms. But the chemistry of joy is not a one-sided phenomenon, in which chemical elements single-handedly affect our mood. Our mental outlook, our spiritual practice, and our understanding of the larger questions of life and self all affect our chemistry as well. Indeed, when we are truly able to achieve joy, we come to see that there is very little distinction among mind, body, and spirit.

TAKE THE BUDDHIST PSYCHOLOGY QUESTIONNAIRE

In Buddhist psychology there are three well-known "types." While our personalities are more complex than that, it may be helpful to find out what your primary tendency is. For each question, circle the answer that best describes you. If more than one answer seems to fit, circle both, or all three.

1. When I get stressed, my first emotional response tends to be:
   a. fear
   b. anger
   c. confusion

2. I worry most about other people:
   a. disliking me
   b. letting me down
   c. abandoning me

3. I have the most trouble tolerating:
   a. uncertainty
   b. disappointment
   c. the need to tell people what I want

4. One of my most noticeable qualities is
   a. sensitivity
   b. ambition and drive
   c. steadiness

5. When I need to confront someone with whom I have a problem, I tend to
   a. meekly ask them to do better
   b. offer strong, sharp criticism
   c. tell myself that it's most likely my problem and try to find something I can do differently

6. I often find myself
   a. worried that I won't have enough of what I need

b. angry with people who are not doing what they should

c. uncertain of what I feel

7. If I could have one wish, it would be to feel
   a. calm and secure
   b. supported and understood
   c. energetic and alive

8. When I feel anxious, upset, or depressed, I tend to
   a. worry
   b. criticize
   c. shut down

9. If my friends or family were asked to name my greatest weakness, they would probably say I'm too
   a. nervous
   b. demanding
   c. hard to read

10. I often feel
    a. unworthy
    b. frustrated
    c. numb

SCORING: Count the number of answers that were:
   a:___ (this corresponds to the Grasping or Fear type)
   b:___ (this corresponds to the Rejecting or Anger type)
   c:___ (this corresponds to the Denial or Adrift type)

If you scored significantly higher in one category, that's your type. If you've got high scores in two categories, you're a combination type. If you've got relatively equal scores in all three categories, you're that rare phenomenon, a three-part combination type.

THE BUDDHIST PSYCHOLOGICAL TYPES

Now that you have a sense of where you fall in this spectrum, let's consider each type more carefully. But remember, each of us contains *all* of these traits—just in different combinations. So read all the chapters in this step without being be too concerned about pigeonholing yourself.

Since I came clean about my Ayurvedic typing, I'll offer the same confession for my Buddhist Emotional type. As you may have guessed from my being a vata, I'm a Fear or Grasping type. Although my own mindfulness practice helps me stay in balance, when I get stressed, I go immediately to a place of "I'm not good enough" or "I'm not going to get the things I need." Fortunately, I'm usually able to rely on one of the techniques in Chapter 15 to help me regain my balance. So as you read through the following profiles, take heart. We all have our default positions, our favorite "unwise strategies," to use the Buddhist term. The good news is that by becoming aware of them, we can make different, better choices.

Grasping or Fear Type

Motto: There's never enough.

Automatic reaction to stress: Always acquire *more*.

When operating from strength and security: Knows when he or she is stressed and takes positive action to do something about it.

When operating from weakness or insecurity: Confuses external or physical satisfaction—through money, food, security, status, or sex—with inner peace.

Western brain-chemistry connection: When depressed, likely to be diagnosed with anxious depression or serotonin depletion; may be helped by dietary and exercise recommendations for serotonin deficiency.

Ayurvedic connection: Corresponds in many ways to Air type, or vata; may be helped by Ayurvedic Mind-Body medicine recommendations for Air types.

Primary Pitfalls:
    insecurity
    fear and anxiety
    difficulty letting go
    scarcity
    envy and greed
    seeking to fill a void
    the feeling that there is never enough

As the name suggests, the Fear-based Emotional type tends to react to stress with fear and anxiety. People in this category have a tendency to *grasp*, to hold tightly to possessions, ideas, other people, or situations. They often have difficulty letting go, even when they see clearly that an idea, person, or situation isn't serving them well.

No matter how much Fear types acquire, however—whether their acquisitions take the form of money, relationships, activities, or information—they tend to be plagued by insecurity and the fear that there is somehow not enough, at least not for them. As a result, they suffer from envy and greed. When you're in a grasping state of mind, satisfaction comes rarely and is then only fleeting. The moment you've tasted the desired fruit, dissatisfaction returns and the wanting begins again.

According to Buddhist psychology, the antidote to the fear of insufficiency is generosity. When you give to others—or to yourself—you realize that you *have* enough and that you *are* enough. Take as your new motto "All is well" and begin to give generously whenever you feel that it is not.

Rejecting or Anger Type

Motto: Whatever I have, it's not good enough.

Automatic reaction to stress: Keep the world at a distance.

When operating from strength and security: Sees clearly when a person, item, or situation is problematic and acts to get rid of it or move away from it.

When operating from weakness and insecurity: Tends to take everything personally, including the weaknesses and shortcomings of loved ones, or random situations that cannot be prevented.

Western brain-chemistry connection: When depressed, likely to be diagnosed with agitated depression or excess of dopamine in relation to serotonin; may be helped by dietary and exercise recommendations for excess dopamine and serotonin deficiency.

Ayurvedic connection: Corresponds in many ways to Fire type, or pitta; may be helped by Ayurvedic Mind-Body medicine recommendations for Fire types.

Primary Pitfalls:
    tendency to push away
    being judgmental

feeling that "nothing is right"
anger
hatred
critical or even destructive of others around them

If Grasping/Fear types tend to cling, Rejecting/Anger types tend to push away people, situations, and opportunities that have disappointed them or that seem to evoke disappointing experiences from the past. Anger types are often filled with judgment: a rejection of things as they are and a wish for them to be different. If you're an out-of-balance Anger type, nothing is ever quite right. Nothing is good enough. Your mind is filled not with what's working or what's making you happy but with what you don't like. You respond to stress with anger, frustration, aggressiveness, and hostility, blaming others, yourself, or both whenever life doesn't work out as planned or desired.

Of course Anger types feel fearful as well. Their response to insecurity, however, is to get angry and, in some cases, even to hate. Life seems to have let them down, and as a result, they're willing to judge the world as failing and punish it accordingly.

What's the solution for Anger types? Buddhist psychologists believe that the antidote to anger is compassion. Learn to see the weakness, fear, and vulnerability in others and in yourself, and to view it with tenderness. Take as your motto that beautiful statement of Buddhist philosopher Thich Nhat Hanh: "Whenever you are angry at someone, remember that he or she is in pain, too."

Adrift or Denial Type

Motto: There's no point in getting upset.
Automatic reaction to stress: Numb out and disconnect from painful feelings.
When operating from strength and security: Can take responsibility for a bad situation, avoiding blame or resentment.
When operating from weakness or insecurity: Tends to allow bad situations to continue far too long because of not being in touch with feelings of anger and sorrow.
Western brain-chemistry connection: When depressed, likely to be diagnosed with melancholia, or extreme sorrow, related to a shortage of

dopamine; may be helped by dietary and exercise recommendations for insufficient norepinephrine/dopamine.

Ayurvedic connection: Corresponds in many ways to Earth type, or kapha; may be helped by Ayurvedic Mind-Body medicine recommendations for Earth types.

Primary Pitfalls:
    denial
    lack of clarity
    flatness or apathy
    sluggishness or lethargy
    psychologically "asleep"

Rather than turning to fear or anger, this Emotional type tends to react to stress with confusion. This is the personality type that, when confronted with a difficult situation, simply "turns off," "numbs out," or freezes, seemingly without either emotions or opinions.

This group has psychologically fallen asleep. They are adrift. If you're in this category, you may be aware of some sadness in your life, but more often you're experiencing a *lack* of feeling, a flatness or apathy frequently accompanied by mental confusion, difficulty making decisions, lethargy, and sluggishness. Instead of feeling angry or fearful, you simply feel befuddled: unsure of how you feel, what you want, or what you'd like to change.

Fear may be at the root of your condition, too—fear of change, of losing a person you care about, of being "a bad person," of your own buried anger. But your response to this fear is your favorite psychological defense—denial.

The antidote to denial is waking up. Let your motto become "I see clearly and accept all that is." It may seem safer to go through life asleep—but only when you awaken can you know joy.

SUFFERING AND SOLUTIONS

Of course we are all familiar with each of these states. But most of us fall into one of these categories more easily than the others. It is our default mode, our "favorite flavor," our habitual response to suffering and stress, even if we act it out in different ways. A Fear type might buy a huge life-insurance policy—or simply surround herself with dependent men who shower her with attention. An Anger type might refuse to marry and maintain few friendships—or form a loyal group of loved ones who are then the subject of intense criticism. And self-delusion comes in many versions: Denial of your feelings, a rose-colored optimism, a determinedly negative self-image are only some of the ways people can set themselves adrift.

The good news is that once we become aware of these patterns, we can begin to adapt new, more effective strategies. The first step is to become mindful and to see the human experience in clear, honest terms. So in the remainder of this chapter, I'll explain the basic principles on which mindfulness is based—a way of looking at suffering, joy, and life itself that I have found extremely helpful in overcoming depression.

SUFFERING IS UNIVERSAL

As the Buddhists say, "All of life is suffering." Buddhists love stories and parables, so here's a famous tale that helps make clear the truth behind this concept.

Kisa Gotami's daughter had died, and she was in agony over the loss. She had heard that the Buddha was capable of miracles, and she went to him, begging for her daughter to be brought back to life. The Buddha felt great compassion for the poor woman and promised he would help her—but only if she could bring him some mustard seed from a home that had known no sorrow.

Filled with hope, Kisa set out on her search. She knew that mustard seed was a common spice, and surely every home in the village had some. But as she knocked on every door, she heard one sad story after another. "Oh, we lost Grandfather last year." "My son was born with a clubfoot and cannot walk." "My mother suffers from palsy and is near death." "I lost two daughters in childbirth and have just miscarried again." Everywhere she went, the story was the same—sorrow, loss, and grief marked every home.

Soon Kisa realized that suffering was universal. No human on earth could escape sorrow and loss. She returned to the Buddha and asked, "What do I do now?" Buddha's precepts for coping with universal suffering touched her heart, and she became one of his earliest and most devoted followers.

I can't believe that Kisa's revelation removed or even diminished her pain. The loss of a child is an irreparable blow, and from what I've seen among patients and friends, I don't believe it ever stops hurting. But I do believe that Kisa's newfound perspective changed her relationship to her pain. Before her understanding deepened, she was anguished and angry. All she could think was how much she wished her child had not died, how much she did not want the world to be as it was. She resisted the blow that life had dealt her, tightening up, hardening herself against it. If she had been a Fear type, she might have been eaten up with envy of other parents whose children had not died. If she'd been an Anger type, she might have railed against the unfairness of life. As a Denial type, she might have shut down, numbed out, blurring her grief into a vague sense of sorrow and loss that she neither fully experienced nor fully released.

Then she grasped that suffering was universal, that what had happened to her, painful as it might be, was an inevitable part of life. I think of her as accepting the blow life dealt her—not fearfully, angrily, or passively, but simply, with all the fullness of her genuine grief. Her pain might continue to throb for the rest of her life—but it no longer determined her thoughts or actions. She found some freedom, and ultimately, some joy—not in spite of her pain, or even because of it, but simply alongside it.

PAIN AND STRESS ARE UNAVOIDABLE; SUFFERING IS OPTIONAL

> You come to me with your problems and hope that
> I can help. You are human. Face that first.
> —IDRIES SHAH, ISLAMIC
> WRITER AND PHILOSOPHER

It is so hard, this human journey. Each of us is subject to all the vulnerabilities, all the moods, the pain, the reactivity, the suffering that comes with being human. Each of us has taken on the challenge of our own personality—our individual sensitivities, our own peculiar insecurities, the things that push our buttons, or stop us short, or shut us down. All of us are prey to the fruitless striving for perfection or the impossible desire to please others.

The poet Rumi has a wonderful line about what it's like to be human: "Every day, we wake up empty and scared." So start by accepting that it's okay to suffer or to feel depressed at times. And then learn to distinguish between the pain that is unavoidable and the suffering that we create for ourselves.

Let me use an example of physical pain to illustrate the extent to which our individual responses affect our experience of the world's pain. Suppose two people are stung by a bee. Both of them feel pain, and certainly neither would say that the bee sting was desirable. But for one person, that's as far as it goes. He notices a little redness and swelling around the sting, he puts some ice on it, and the pain goes away. In an hour or so, he's forgotten all about it.

For the second person, the bee sting is the beginning of a nightmare. This person is allergic to bees, and her body reacts to bee venom far beyond the actual danger of the sting. An enormous redness and swelling spreads swiftly from the bee sting outward. Her immune system pulls out all the stops, and soon her lungs swell, too, and she has trouble breathing. Her body is only trying to save her from what it perceives as a terrifying threat—but her response to the pain might actually kill her. Only an injection of rapid-acting antihistamine or an immune-system suppressant will save her from dying as a result of a seemingly minor insult.

Note that the type and amount of bee venom is the same in both people. But their bodies' reactions to the sting can make the difference between a trivial pain and a life-threatening bout of suffering.

Just as we have different responses to pain, so do we have different responses to stress and abuse. One person thrives on the challenge of a demanding job, while the next crumbles beneath its weight. One person forgives his tormentors, while the next is destroyed by the bitterness and hatred that seem to last forever—causing her far greater suffering than the abusive act that engendered the pain in the first place. One person is somehow enlarged by an encounter with depression, while the next is markedly diminished by it.

As we saw in Chapter 2, we seem to be born with certain tendencies—to fret or to relax, to turn quickly to fear or to remain steady in our confidence, to spring to anger on a hair trigger or to blithely forgive and forget. But beyond our genetic makeup, we've *learned* to react, automatically and unconsciously, to life's little stresses and insults, and just as with the person allergic to bee stings, our reactions do more damage than the initial source of pain. So regardless of our temperament or bio-chemical "givens," our job is to change our automatic and destructive *reactions* into conscious and healthy *responses*.

In this way, suffering is optional, although pain—both physical and emotional—is not. Even if we live in constant pain, we have a choice about whether or not to suffer with it. Although thoughts and feelings will arise, seemingly of their own accord ("I feel miserable"; "Why does this happen to me?"; "I wish I were more like So-and-so"), we can choose to focus on those thoughts and feelings, to feed them with our attention—or we can choose to let them pass while we focus on other things.

WHAT WE FOCUS UPON, GROWS

Take a moment now to do an exercise. Give yourself a few quiet min-utes where you will be undisturbed. Set this book down, take a pad and pen, and set them next to you. Close your eyes, take a few calming breaths, and invite your imagination to engage. Reflect for a few mo-ments upon what you are like when you are most alive, most joyous, most truly your best self. Whom are you with? What are you doing? How do you look and feel? See yourself in your mind's eye as joyous and present, and allow yourself to experience this feeling now, as best you can. Then take some time to write about what you imagined and what you learned from it.

Now repeat the exercise, only this time reflect upon what you are like when you are at your worst: depressed, moody, unable to handle the stresses of daily life. Again, try to see yourself in as much detail as possi-ble. Whom are you with? What are you doing? How do you look and feel? See yourself as stressed and miserable, and allow yourself to experi-ence this feeling, now, as best you can. Again, write down your experi-ence.

Now ask yourself how the second experience was different from the first? Which do you prefer?

I'd like you to notice how, with just a few minutes' effort, you were able to create two very different experiences for yourself. Nothing in your life had actually changed, except that you'd read a few more sen-tences of this book. No loved ones had abandoned you, no work problems arose, no opportunities for happiness or security had been lost. Yet you were able to take yourself from a joyous or at least a calm state into a state of misery and depression—simply with the power of your mind. Although you don't do it consciously or "on purpose," if you're often depressed, your mind follows a similar course several times a day, so start becoming aware of the thoughts, feelings, and experiences on which you choose to focus.

This can be a very difficult point for many of us to grasp. When we're in the depths of our depression, nothing is more insulting—or less helpful—than hearing someone say, "It's your own fault. Why don't you just buck up and think of something cheerful?" When you're overwhelmed with a flood of fear, anger, or confusion, you *know* that's all there is. You can't begin to imagine that life holds calm, compassion, joy.

I promise you, whatever you feel, however deep your depression runs, you *can* experience joy within it and alongside it. If you've already begun to act on some of the diet, exercise, and lifestyle suggestions in Steps One and Two, you may already have begun to feel a bit better. But beyond these important physical steps, there are mental, emotional, and spiritual steps you can take as well, not to eradicate the automatic reactions you've practiced for so long, but to train yourself to turn to new responses. Just as you've learned to focus on the "worst-self" aspects of your experience—a focus aided and abetted by your brain chemistry and genetics, to be sure—now you can learn to create that "best-self" experience for yourself, simply by practicing it over and over again.

I'll share with you one final story to illustrate the importance of where we place our attention. This one comes not from the East but from our own North America, a lovely Native American tale about a boy and his grandfather:

> A young boy, about five years old, goes to spend the summer with his grandfather, who is a respected tribal elder. He adores his grandfather and watches his every move. Very quickly he notices a pattern. Every morning, about sunrise, his grandfather goes to an altar in his home, takes off a necklace, and places it on the altar. Then he sits in silence for several minutes. Afterward, he puts on the necklace and continues with his day. Every evening, around sunset, he repeats this ritual.
>
> After a few days, the little boy can no longer contain himself. "Grandfather, what are you doing?" he asks.

"I am taking some time to quiet my spirit and honor our ancestors," the old man replies.

"But what is on the necklace?" the boy inquires.

The grandfather takes off the necklace and shows it to the boy. On it are the heads of two wolves.

"Grandfather, what do they mean?"

"Well," the grandfather replies, "inside each of us there are two wolves fighting to control us. One of them is scared and mean and has a hunger that can never be filled. It cares only about itself. The other is brave and kind and shares whatever it has with others. It cares as much about the community as it does for itself."

Wide-eyed and a little frightened, the boy asks, "Grandfather, which wolf will win?"

The old man smiles at his grandson. "Whichever one we feed the most."

12

FEAR TYPES:
ALWAYS GRASPING AFTER MORE

If you met my patient Joe, you would never think of him as greedy. A tall, thin man with a shy smile, Joe is quick to hold the door for the person behind him, eager to volunteer for the jobs nobody else wants at his local parent–teacher association, the kind of guy who'll come over in forty-below weather to help a neighbor jump-start his car. People who know Joe would call him unselfish—even generous.

But Joe's life is ruled by a strong sense of insufficiency, the belief that there is not enough and that *he* is not enough. This perception of scarcity and lack is the greatest source of unhappiness for Fear types, which is why the Buddhist term for this category is "grasping." If you believe you're "not enough," you'll always grasp for more.

Let's look at how this works for Joe. He's been employed for the past fifteen years at a local social-service agency, a job he usually enjoys. But when he gets caught up in his sense of insufficiency, his mind becomes unsettled and he tends to fret. Regret, wanting, and worry dominate his thoughts. He loses his access to the present moment because he's focused on the past—things he did or didn't do that might have given him more of what he desires now. I call it the "if-only" mind: "If only I'd taken that job in Minneapolis," "If only I'd gotten a different degree," "If only I'd put aside more money last year." Life in the present begins to seem worthless, because of something that did or didn't happen in the past.

Sometimes Joe loses his contact with the present in a different way: through worries about the future. This is also an "if-only" mind, but focused on wanting something that he believes might make him feel satisfied and secure later on. "If only I had money for that European vacation," "If only my wife weren't complaining all the time," "If only I were a braver person, ready to leave this job and take a better one."

Besides the "if-only" mind, Joe struggles with a "what-if" mind—another way of focusing on the future at the expense of the present. "What if the stock market doesn't bounce back before my kids go to college?" "What if my marriage doesn't recover from this rough patch and goes completely sour?" "What if my depression doesn't go away?"

On a good day, Joe can recognize these thoughts for what they are and brush them aside. But when he's stressed, out of balance, and vulnerable to depression, his fleeting tendency to regret might be harder to dismiss. His mind seizes on the "if-only" thoughts and responds with a powerful wave of envy, greed, and insecurity: "I'm such a timid guy. Why can't I be more like my brother William? He's always ready to take a chance—and look what a great life *he* has." "My kids are great—but I want them to go to the best schools, and I'll never be able to afford that on my salary. If only I had more money." "If only my wife understood me better. If only I'd married someone warmer and more open."

Eventually, these thoughts and feelings begin to feed on themselves, much in the manner of compound interest. From being only a small part of Joe's mental and emotional life, they grow exponentially with every moment of attention he gives them. Soon the depression takes the familiar turn of self-questioning, self-doubt, and even self-hatred. "I'm such a loser. Why can't I be more successful? I'm letting everybody down. Other people are so much better than I am. No wonder my wife isn't interested in me. . . . No wonder my kids don't respect me. . . ." Before he knows it, Joe is mired in the depths of depression, struggling against a sense of insufficiency and lack that seems far bigger than he is, grasping for something—anything—that might give him the security and peace he seeks.

THE POWER OF THE BUSY MIND

Although he can't always make use of his knowledge, Joe would be the first to admit that most of his problems start right in his own mind. This is not to say that he's "making everything up." He may have genuine problems that need his attention or that he may never be able to solve. But he also has trouble distinguishing between reality and what he believes about reality.

For example, Joe has no idea, really, of what his kids' future will be. He can make a good guess, an informed prediction, about how much college is likely to cost, what he's likely to be able to afford, and how available financial aid may be. But he doesn't really *know* what the future will bring, nor how he and his kids will feel about it when it arrives. If concern over his kids' college tuition leads him to take useful action—putting money away, researching financial aid, helping his kids get good grades—then his mind has done a good job of identifying problems and developing solutions. But if Joe's perception of potential problems produces endless fretting, which in turn leads to fear, insecurity, and self-hatred, then his mind has led him astray.

All of us wish, to some extent, that we could control the future. We'd like to believe that if we do the right things and avoid the wrong ones, we can guarantee health and safety for ourselves and our loved ones. In one way, this wish is a good thing: The desire to protect our survival often leads us to take useful actions.

But in another way, our wish for control creates a dangerous illusion. In fact, we have no idea what the future holds. We can't ever be sure how our actions will affect our future. Maybe the money we wisely invested will be lost in the stock market, while the silly hobby we took up on impulse turns into a million-dollar career. That doesn't mean we should stop saving money or pursue frivolous pipe dreams. But it does mean that we shouldn't waste time feeling anxious or insufficient, wishing we could control a future that will take its own course.

It's bad enough when our minds simply generate thoughts—"What if this happens?" "Why didn't that happen?" But beyond simply registering information—real or imaginary—our minds tend to add a quality or feeling tone to every experience. A job with lots of money is *good*, a broken heart is *bad*. Being able to care for our children is *good*, letting them down is *bad*.

Again, this filtering of our experiences has a useful aspect. If we didn't pursue pleasure and avoid pain, how would we ensure our own survival? The problem comes not because our minds make these judgments, but because we overvalue them. If we think something is bad, it must *be* bad—and then we cause ourselves a lot of unnecessary suffering by worrying about it, fearing it, regretting it, or resenting it.

Here's another Buddhist parable to illustrate my point:

A farmer had a beautiful stallion that he used to plow his fields. One day, the horse ran away. "That's too bad," the neighbors said, but the farmer simply shrugged.

Then the runaway horse returned, bringing with him a wild mare he had found. The mare was pregnant, and soon the farmer had three horses where before he had only one. "That's great!" the neighbors said, but the farmer simply shrugged.

The mare gave birth to a new little colt, and when the time came, the farmer's only son began to train the horse. One day, the colt bucked so hard he threw the farmer's son onto the ground and broke the son's back. Now the son was crippled and could not walk. "That's too bad," the neighbors said, but the farmer simply shrugged.

Then a war broke out, and the army came and took all the boys in the village off to fight. Eventually, they were all killed in battle. But the farmer's son, because of his injuries, was spared and allowed to remain at home. "Lucky you," the neighbors said, but the farmer simply shrugged. . . .

As you can see, life takes many twists and turns. Impossible to know what apparently good fortune will turn bad, what seemingly hard luck will become our greatest blessing. Impossible, too, to escape the sorrows of life: Everyone in the farmer's story undergoes some form of pain, and no one is granted enough knowledge to prevent it. Only the farmer, while experiencing pain, avoids suffering. He accepts what life brings him without judging—not without *feeling*, but without judging.

TRYING TO FILL THE VOID

Although in theory we can always choose to stop suffering, often most of us don't. Why not? One reason is that we have a mistaken idea about what will bring us happiness. We are all prone to think that we could overcome our insecurity if only we could fill the void that we sometimes fear is at the center of our lives.

Of course insecurity is part of life, and when we can accept that fact, we can become truly secure. But we're far more prone to try to *do* something to overcome our insecurity, to buy an expensive object or distract ourselves with an endless round of parties or bury our fears in a new romance. Although I'm supposed to "know better," I'm just as guilty in this regard as anyone else. All too often, instead of accepting my discomfort and letting it pass, I find myself struggling mightily against it. On my best days, I do my best to achieve the goals I think are right—and then I relax and accept whatever the outcome actually is. On my not-so-good days, I, too, greet "failure" with anger, resentment, envy, and the rest. At least I've finally learned that when these feelings arise, the solution is not to ignore them or to blame myself for having them. The solution is simply to feel them and let them pass. That may be easier said than done—but it is the road to joy, especially for Fear types.

THE TRAP OF UNWORTHINESS

Joe's problem was less a conscious desire for "more" than a tendency to feel inadequate and unworthy. For him, the currency in shortest supply was love. Although he knew on some level that both his wife and his two children loved him, he often had trouble experiencing their feelings for him. Instead, he felt lonely, abandoned, and unworthy—and he blamed himself for the barren world in which he lived.

Over the years of working with me, Joe learned that the first signal for his depressive spiral was any twinge of envy. The lower he felt, the more he tended to elevate others, envying their happiness, their relationships, their character, and ultimately their greater worth. He couldn't help feeling that if they got what they wanted, he had less chance of getting "his."

Of course, when Joe and I spoke directly about these issues, Joe insisted that he had no conscious wish to deprive anyone of anything. But at an unconscious level, Joe was ruled by what Buddhist psychologists would call the "wanting mind." Somewhere deep inside, Joe was certain that he simply wasn't good enough, and he desired something, anything, to fill the void inside.

THE HOLD OF THE PAST

Although I believe our ultimate goal is to live every moment fully in the present, I also know that sometimes, in order to understand the present, we have to visit the past. For Joe—as for many other Fear types—the issues that underlay his insecure grasping were rooted in childhood experiences of betrayal.

When I first began working with him, Joe recalled his childhood in a mostly happy light. But when he was still very young, his father had left the family for reasons that Joe didn't understand. Although Joe got along well with his stepfather after his parents divorced, this early abandonment by his biological father left a powerful legacy.

Now, whenever Joe began to feel depressed, he was vaguely aware of something lurking just below the surface, something heavy that seemed to weigh him down. Although Joe talked relatively easily about this childhood trauma, he had a harder time acknowledging how much anger and insecurity he still felt as a result. "Sure, my father left us. But I don't need to take it personally. And I sure don't need to let it affect me for my entire life!"

Yet, as we explored this issue, Joe began to see that his father's abandonment had done just that. All his life, Joe had been carrying unresolved feelings of abandonment and rejection, feelings that he'd buried at the time because they seemed too powerful and overwhelming to the five-year-old boy who'd had to deal with them. His adult mind understood that Joe's father hadn't left because of *him*. But the five-year-old Joe blamed himself, as all children tend to do. Because he had never seen the issue clearly or been willing to reexperience the grief, he had never quite realized how powerful it was.

SMALL SELF, BIG SELF

One way of describing Joe's problem is that his inner life was dominated by his "smaller self," the individual ego within each of us whose only job is to guarantee our survival. In Buddhist psychology, we all have both a smaller and a larger self. The smaller self is the part of ourselves that has a history, a "story" that we hold on to at all costs. "My father left me when I was five," or "I was sexually abused in my teens," or "I have always had trouble getting into good relationships." It's not so much that this story isn't true or even that it isn't important—but when we are in our small selves, we tend to think that this story is all there is.

Because our small self is entirely focused on self-preservation, it tends to be dominated by fear: of not getting enough, not *being* enough, getting hurt, encountering the unknown, making a mistake, not being liked, displeasing others, undergoing change—you name it. Our small self fears anything that *might* threaten our survival—and it is sure that any changed circumstance or new idea will do just that. Like an over-protective parent, it wants to keep us safe and isolated from anything it can't completely control.

Unfortunately, this endless search for security won't create a happy, fulfilled life. It won't even make us *feel* safe. As long as we stay locked inside our small self, we're guaranteed to fear everything that remains outside—that is, everything. To identify with this small self is to ensure that we will suffer.

Fortunately for us, there is a larger self on which we might choose to focus. Have you ever felt a moment of true transcendence? Perhaps you were looking up at the stars, or sitting in a church or synagogue. Maybe you were with a person—friend, family member, or lover—whom you truly loved, who you knew truly loved you. Or perhaps you had just solved a pressing problem, completed some work of which you were proud, or just woken up feeling good. However you found your moment of peace—through nature, solitude, prayer, companionship, or work—at that moment, you felt large, whole, connected. You felt a sense of un-shakable peace and security, as though you were finally complete. At that moment, you went beyond the bounds of your small self and found a larger understanding of who you are, a person connected to the natu-ral world, the divine, and all humanity.

If you have ever felt this type of transcendence, you need to know that you can always re-create it for yourself, remembering who you truly are and where joy truly resides. If you've never had an experience like this, don't despair. The practices I share with you in Chapter 15 will prime you for just such feelings, and you'll learn that you can repeat the experience as often as you like. That's not because I know some magic formula, but because this larger self *is* as true as our smaller self—truer—even if we're often blind to it. And once you've experienced this larger self, you'll learn to seek the feeling in your daily life as well as through the exercises I'll suggest.

Although we don't talk about it much in Western society, people find transcendence—a connection to something larger—in all sorts of places: religion, politics, work, love, even at a sports game, where for one shining moment you share your team's victory with ten thousand other people and feel connected to every one of them. You can also find transcendence in those small, private moments when you give or receive kindness—when the counter guy smiles at you while handing you your coffee, or when you hold the door for a woman burdened with packages and hear her grateful "thank you." Somehow, you and another person—friend or stranger—have made a connection through love and compassion, and this connection reminds you of who you really are.

Joe liked the distinction between the small, false self and the larger, true self, because it made room for the parts of himself that he didn't like so much. Now he didn't have to think of his insecurities or his envy as wrong or bad. He could think of them as simply less skilled or less wise responses, reactions that came from a smaller, less complete place. Instead of berating himself for his shortcomings, he could simply acknowledge that he had different ways of operating—which he could expect to result in different outcomes. Instead of trying to change himself—which implied a judgment that there was something wrong with him—he could simply work to become more aware—more *mindful*, in Buddhist terms—of what he was feeling and how he was acting. He could decide, too, which self to feed, his small self or his larger one.

DETACHING FROM THE SMALLER SELF

Half of any person is wrong and weak and off the beaten path. Half!
The other half is dancing and swimming and flying in the invisible joy!
—RUMI

As these lines from a Rumi poem suggest, we are more than just a walking bag of insecurities, small selves, problems, symptoms, or illness. Much more. But how do we coax ourselves into the larger self, where all that invisible joy resides?

The first step is to remember that being human isn't bad. It's just incomplete. No matter how much we yearn for the joy and contentment of our larger selves, as long as we're on this earth, we're going to have times of slipping back into the insecurity of our smaller selves. I love the Rumi poem because it reminds me that all of us are both strong and weak, large and small, whole and unwhole. And so we can choose to focus on our best, largest, and most alive selves—while not despairing at the continued existence of our smaller selves.

So Joe had to realize that he was continually feeding his own pain by the kinds of thoughts he was reinforcing within himself, the core beliefs to which he clung. He began to see how competitive he was, how his first response to a friend's happiness was pain, envy, and anxiety. It hurt Joe to hear about one friend's sudden growth and transformation, another's involvement with an exciting new relationship, and a third's success at work. "I guess every time someone else gets some good news, I feel like they're gaining on me," Joe admitted. He saw another's victory as his own defeat—and the price of defeat seemed to be the loss of his very self.

As we worked further, Joe's understanding became more specific. It wasn't so much that he thought he'd lose his identity as that he'd stop being "special," "the only one." Of course, in one sense, every single one of us is unique and special. But Joe was used to seeing his specialness in terms of others' lack. If he was smart, then someone else had to be stupid. If he was successful, someone else had failed. This put a terrible price on Joe's success, for every time he felt happy, he had also to feel the guilt that came from being happy at another's expense. And then whenever a loved one or even a stranger enjoyed a measure of happiness, Joe felt—unconsciously—that it came at *his* expense.

This process of self-awareness has its dangers. As Joe learned things he didn't like about himself and his core beliefs, he risked falling into an even deeper depression. Now that he knew how involved he was with negative core beliefs, how many negative qualities he was feeding, he might feel even worse about himself than he did before. But I encouraged Joe to be easy with himself, to hold these insights lightly and not grasp on to them with his smaller self. If he could embrace this insight instead of resisting it, then, like the woman who had lost her child, he could begin to see that *all* of us suffer from the power of our smaller selves, that *all* of us, as Rumi said, are at least halfway wrong and weak and off the beaten path. Even Joe's suffering and smallness could be a bridge to link him to the rest of humanity.

Ultimately, becoming more aware of his flaws enabled Joe to accept them—and then move beyond them. He came to understand that while he—like the rest of us—will always be an envious, grasping person, he could *also*—like the rest of us—always be generous, giving, and secure, "dancing in the invisible joy."

13

ANGER TYPES: NEVER SATISFIED

Rick was an angry man—a *very* angry man. He was referred to me by his therapist to assess whether medication could help his depression. Normally, we associate depression with being unhappy, and Rick was definitely unhappy—miserable even. He couldn't sleep, had little energy, and thought a lot about suicide. But although his diagnosis was depression, his predominant mood was anger, the kind that could burn you if you got in its way.

Rick had already seen and rejected nearly a dozen therapists, most of them within the first session. His list of complaints against them was endless: They didn't listen well, failed to take his problems seriously enough, charged too much money, offered gimmicky suggestions. Rick found reasons to reject each of his therapists as easily as he rejected almost everyone else in his life. In fact, he was about to leave his current therapist—the one who had recommended him to me—although he had been seeing him for only a few months.

THE SMALL SELF OF JUDGMENT

Rick was clearly a Rejecting or Anger type, what Buddhist psychology terms an Aversion type. Filled with anger, his was an energy of pushing away, of rejecting even those people, opportunities, and situations that he most desired. Rick was still in his early forties, too young to worry about the heart disease that so often plagues people with this temperament. But one could say that Rick already had a disease of the heart. From my point of view, he was slowly but surely destroying himself from within.

Rick was attached to his small self—so strongly attached to it that he wore it like a second skin. Unlike Joe, he wasn't concerned with insufficiency but with inadequacy, so that his mind was completely caught up in seeing what was wrong with everything. Rick was a prime example of the "judging mind," the mind that continually criticizes and rejects what is. Whereas the what-if mind sees the world in terms of what it *wants*, the judging mind looks for what it *dislikes* and can *reject*.

Unlike the what-if mind, the judging mind has little interest in either the past or future. Instead, it's preoccupied with the here and now. But because its relationship to the present is one of constant criticism, the judging mind actually prevents Anger types from experiencing their lives moment by moment. Anger types have difficulty abandoning themselves to the experience of, say, watching a movie, dating a woman, or working at their chosen job because of the way they distance themselves through their constant evaluations and judgments: "I don't like that movie. . . . I'm disappointed with this woman. . . . I can't stand where I work."

Having registered its dislike, the Angry mind goes on to find a reason for it: "The movie was too dull . . . She doesn't give me enough attention. . . . This job pays too little for what I have to put up with." Now that the judgment has been not only made but also substantiated, Anger types can forget about finding any pleasure in whatever has been rejected. And they can certainly forget about being surprised, engaged, or even caught off guard. The extraordinary uncertainty of experience—the way it changes from moment to moment, the way it transforms *us*—can be pushed away. All experiences can be kept at a safe distance, while Anger types' judgments and reasons provide them with the illusion of control.

Sadly, Anger types are rarely aware of their own behavior and its effects on others—or on themselves. They almost never realize how quickly they write people off, how rapidly they dismiss unfamiliar ideas or reject new possibilities. On a date, for example, instead of staying open to the possibility that a woman might change as you get to know her, that a man might behave differently under different circumstances, that people are an unpredictable mixture of good and bad to whom we may have a wide range of reactions and responses, Anger types jump to their judgments, often without realizing the part they themselves have played in the encounter. For example, an Anger type might find it difficult to imagine that the woman he dated was nervous precisely because he himself was so critical and judgmental. "She's just too awkward," Rick might say dismissively about a woman he'd gone out with, without realizing that perhaps his own negative attitude had helped to bring out that particular side of his date.

Likewise, Anger types might not realize their own stake in the judgments they make. It was far easier for Rick to say something like "She's way too insistent about that topic," or "Doesn't she see how wrong she is?" than to pause and reflect, "That topic really pushes my buttons" or "I feel very strongly about that issue."

In fact, Rick was letting his fear run his life—not the fear of insufficiency that haunted Joe, but the fear of being attacked or diminished. Every time Rick even imagined that an attack might come, he responded with an instant blast of aggression that made it extremely hard to get close to him. Sadly, Rick had no idea of his own role in this dynamic. If he could have realized how often people left his presence with hurt feelings or the sense of being humiliated, he would have been astonished. In his own eyes, he was only the victim, the one whom "nobody liked."

FINDING THE TROUBLE WITHIN

As I've worked with Anger types over the years, I'm struck by how quick they are to blame others—and how unaware they can be about their own role in conflicts. Rick, as we've seen, is a prime example, but my patient Joanne was another. Joanne was a woman in her early fifties who had founded her own small business nearly twenty years earlier. She consulted me for some executive coaching sessions because she was frustrated by the way she kept losing employees. She could always find good people, she told me, but just as she got them trained and up to speed, they seemed to leave, despite the excellent salaries she was paying and the good benefits she was offering as well.

I was surprised to hear Joanne's complaints because I'd actually known her by reputation before she ever came to see me. By all accounts, she was a brilliant woman who had built her company from the ground up and was still involved in all aspects of her business. She was energetic, creative, and hard-driving—all considered desirable traits for the American entrepreneur. It wasn't in Joanne's nature to look to herself as the cause of her workplace unhappiness. But that is exactly where we had to go.

Joanne's company was fairly small—only about twenty-five employees, all told, and all of them had a lot of contact with her. I met most of them, and saw them as good, solid people. It didn't take me much time to realize that it was Joanne herself who was driving them out, not with low pay or long hours, but with her relentless criticism and judgment, followed by her need to micromanage even the smallest detail. She spent most of her time telling each of her workers exactly what he or she was doing wrong. No wonder people left as soon as they could.

Joanne finally had to face her own role in the problem when one of her most trusted employees resigned. She was shocked to receive his letter of resignation, which to her came as a complete surprise, and called him into her office for an explanation. Because of their close relationship, the man was willing to tell Joanne what no one else had dared to say: Her constant criticism and rejection of other people's ideas had finally gotten to him. Although he knew that she thought highly of him, he still found her denigrating remarks painful, and he'd started developing migraines and indigestion in response.

Joanne was shocked to think that she had actually helped to make this man sick. We began discussing her Anger-type reactions in a more honest and thoughtful way, and Joanne started to practice some of the heart-opening exercises described in Chapter 15. She also began thinking more deeply about her own experiences with being criticized and rejected. Her father had been a demanding taskmaster, never satisfied and always quick with a sharp remark. Joanne began to realize how much of his negative attitudes and contemptuous responses she had unconsciously adopted.

Joanne's progress was slow, and people have continued to leave her company at a rate she finds distressing. But she's taken the first steps on her road to self-awareness—a small beginning, but a beginning nonetheless.

SEEKING SOLUTIONS IN ALL THE WRONG PLACES

Rick and Joanne shared a trait that is all too common—the wish to blame others for the problems we create ourselves. When we're undergoing stress, our minds automatically go into search mode, seeking reasons why we feel so awful. Unfortunately, we rarely look in the right place—at our own attachment to the small self, our own insistence on feeding our fear, envy, resentment, and confusion. Instead, we seek our answers in the shortcomings we see around us. We may even be right in our judgments. But if we don't also look at our own role in a problem, we'll never come up with a strategy that will really work.

A particularly ineffective strategy that most of us use from time to time is *projection*, the attribution of qualities or motivations to others without sufficient basis in fact. One of my favorite jokes contains a wonderfully extreme example of projection—the certainty that we know what's going on in other people's minds and the willingness to act accordingly:

Levy was miserable. He lay sleepless in his bed in his tiny Lower East Side tenement and watched the snow come down. "Everything happens to me," he thought. "I've just gotten settled into this apartment, and the landlord says I have to move tomorrow. Fine, I'll move—and I've even found another place, right down the block. But now it's snowing, and tomorrow the sidewalks will be full of ice and snow. How will I get my stuff from here to there in this terrible weather?"

Suddenly Levy had a wonderful thought: His friend Goldberg owned a sled. "Wonderful!" he said to himself. "Tomorrow, I'll go over and borrow the sled. I'll load it up with all my possessions and drag it down the street—problem solved!"

Levy was just about to fall asleep when he had a troubling thought. *"What if Goldberg won't lend the sled?"*

"That's ridiculous!" he said to himself. "He's my best friend. He'll be happy to do me a favor. Stop worrying, and go to sleep."

But the thought wouldn't go away. *"What if Goldberg won't lend the sled?"*

"Nonsense," Levy said to himself. "Haven't I always helped him when he needed it? Why, I'm the one who got him his first job. I've even lent him money. Besides, he's a generous guy. Stop worrying and go to sleep."

But once again, the thought returned. *"What if Goldberg won't lend the sled?"*

"The rotten ingrate!" Levy said to himself. "Haven't I always gone out of my way for *him?* And when his son was sick, didn't I stay with the boy for an entire weekend? Doesn't he know I'd do anything for him? And now he won't even lend me his lousy five-dollar sled?"

Enraged, Levy jumped out of bed, threw on his overcoat and galoshes over his pajamas and bare feet, and stalked across the street to Goldberg's apartment. He banged loudly on the door until a befuddled Goldberg, still half-asleep, slowly appeared in the doorway.

"Goldberg!" said Levy in righteous indignation. "You know what you can do with your no-good sled? You and that sled can go straight to hell!" And leaving the astonished Goldberg behind him, Levy stalked back to his own apartment, threw off his snow-covered overcoat and galoshes, and slept the sleep of the just.

I love this story because it makes the concept of projection so clear. Levy is so ready to get angry, to blame others for their supposed shortcomings, to attribute unkind motives to his friend, that he can't even see that he's invented the entire conflict. I like to imagine him telling the story to his other friends the next day, describing in glorious detail Goldberg's selfish refusal, which in his mind has taken on the status of unassailable fact. The story is funny because it's exaggerated, of course. But when I think of the way we get caught up in our own projections, I wonder if the events are exaggerated all that much.

While we're pretty much all guilty of projection, the kinds of projections we make tend to vary based on our type. A Fear type like Joe usually creates projections based on his wishes or fears. If he's feeling envious, he may convince himself that other people are happier, more successful, or simply better than they really are. Or, to soothe his envy, he may imagine that they're somehow worse. Either way, he'll be viewing others through the lens of his own wishes, not as their true selves.

Anger types, by contrast, often tend to project their judgment or blame onto others. "My employees are so ungrateful," Joanne might say. "My business would be so much more successful if Terry were a more reliable employee." Indeed, Joanne is the one who is not grateful to her employees for their hard work on her company's behalf. Instead of seeing this quality in herself, she projects it onto others—and blames the others accordingly.

THE FALSE SEARCH FOR SAFETY

I wasn't able to see Rick for regular therapy, but he sensed with me an acceptance he hadn't found with any of his previous therapists and asked if I'd agree to see him occasionally. After we'd seen each other a few times, he told me what he considered the source of his problems.

When Rick was nine, his family was invited to another family's cabin for a weekend. The other family had a thirteen-year-old son whom Rick liked and looked up to. The two boys were assigned to the same bedroom for the weekend, and that first night, the older boy initiated sexual contact. Confused and not knowing what else to do, Rick allowed the encounter to proceed. But he felt violated, ashamed, and unsafe, and he had no idea how to respond.

Ultimately, he did nothing. He allowed the boy to repeat the encounter the second night, and he said nothing about the incident to anyone. For his entire childhood, adolescence, and young adulthood, he pushed the entire experience, along with the flood of feelings that it had produced, down into the subterranean levels of his psyche. Although consciously he could barely remember the incident, Rick developed the subconscious belief that his own weakness and submissiveness—which he felt had left him open to the first incident—might make him vulnerable to future violations as well.

Rick also unconsciously blamed his parents for not knowing about the problem and protecting him, and he harbored an enormous anger because they had failed him so badly. Rick felt bewildered and alone— and that made him angry.

Because Rick had refused to think about the incident consciously for so many years, he was stuck with a nine-year-old's understanding of what had happened. His young mind had come to the following conclusion: "Either I'm submissive and risk being attacked, or I'm dominant and therefore safe." If that was the choice, Rick decided unconsciously, he'd go for dominance. Certainly, no one else could be relied on to protect him, so he'd have to be ready to protect himself.

In his forties, Rick carried those memories more heavily than ever, along with the bitter feelings that went with them. He'd now had a lifetime of responding to the world based on that incident, a lifetime of feeling like a victim. Ironically, although he wasn't responsible for what had happened to him as a child, he had become responsible for how that incident had affected him. Every day—every hour—Rick was choosing to feed his small self, the self of anger, judgments, and bitterness. He was continuing to follow the choices he had made as a nine-year-old, when he'd decided to shut out others who couldn't be relied on, to respond with anger and aggression when anyone tried to get close.

The nine-year-old Rick had made these choices innocently and unconsciously, not knowing how greatly they'd affect him over the years. His job now was to bring those choices into the light of awareness, realizing that when we make choices unconsciously, we actually lose the power of choice. And the price for losing that power can be enormous.

THE COSTS OF AGGRESSION

The first step for Rick was to realize that although his deepest desires were for intimacy, affection, and love, his own actions were keeping him at arm's length from anyone who might provide him with these creature comforts. For Rick, as for most Anger types, rejection served to insulate him from a supposedly dangerous world.

Based on the past thirty years, Rick had plenty of evidence that every one of his relationships would eventually go terribly wrong. "If it's going to happen sooner or later," he reasoned unconsciously, "why not make it sooner? If I reject first, then I can't be rejected."

All of us may respond to the fear of being hurt by wrapping ourselves in layers of protection. Even if we haven't chosen such an isolated life as Rick's, we may still be keeping our loved ones from ever truly reaching us, or distancing ourselves unnecessarily from the day-to-day joys of life. A hard heart, a bristly personality, an attachment to strength, or a fiercely competitive spirit might mask our fears of closeness and our sense of our own vulnerability. Complete dominance seems to offer at least some protection from the humiliation of losing, the shame of being second best, the vulnerability that comes from being "less" than another. Even when we compete against ourselves, our drive to be "the best" can be a way of keeping us isolated, both from loved ones and from our own experience.

Of course strength, competence, self-protection, and even competition can all be wonderful things. But only when they're conscious choices, made with goodwill. We need only to look at the daily paper to see the costs of untamed aggression. What damage is done to the emerging self-image of a group of boys on a football team that loses by seventy points to a far superior team? What lessons are taught to the twelve-year-old hockey players when the game ends and the fathers of opposing teammates get into a fistfight over one of the ref's controversial calls? What potential is lost when an aspiring graduate student is publicly humiliated by her professor in an unnecessary display of the professor's intellectual superiority?

Aggression breeds aggression, just as violence breeds violence. When we react aggressively—even out of our own fear—we can be sure that the effects of our actions will live on in another. We can see the effects of aggression, violence, and hatred grow and spread—in the Middle East, in Iraq, in the Sudan, in the inner cities, in once-innocent schools across America. This violence did not arise out of nowhere and all at once. It began, in every instance, within human hearts that were, at some time in the past, threatened or violated. In response, a decision was made, consciously or not, to harden that heart, to be strong, to retaliate, to "fight fire with fire." That decision, like the actions that prompted it, made the situation even worse: Every person who decides to add their own anger or hatred to the fire only gives it more fuel to burn. And now the fires of violence are raging, everywhere we turn.

AGGRESSION, POWER, AND LOVE

Although I was only meeting with Rick every few weeks, he was deeply committed to our sessions. He let me know how much it meant to him to feel accepted by me just as he was. "All my other therapists tried to fix me," he told me once. But with me, he didn't feel judged or analyzed or in need of fixing. He felt instead that I was simply sitting with calm acceptance—and that created an opening for him, a place where he finally felt safe.

In fact, I liked Rick. He was bright, articulate, honest, sincere. I could see through the anger, could see the tenderness and longing and the deep desire for freedom and happiness that he kept well hidden most of the time. Although he could not accept himself, I was able to accept him fully, his small self as well as his large. And because I could see that larger self—because I could see more in Rick than he could see in himself—his healing began.

Of course I was Rick's therapist, and I'd had years of training in sitting with calm acceptance. But any of us can create this kind of safe space for another, simply by refraining from judging, by refusing to reject the angry person even though he or she seems to invite it. This acceptance is a gift that can be offered by anyone who has the willingness and whose own heart is still alive.

Think of a small child who is having a tantrum. If you've ever been with a kicking, screaming child who calls out insults and says she hates you, you may know firsthand how tempting it is to retaliate, to get angry, to punish. "Well, I hate you, too!" I've been tempted to say to my own children, on more than one occasion.

But there is certainly another, more tender part of any loving adult who simply sees the innocence in that ranting child and knows that a forceful response will serve neither the adult's nor the child's best interest. Yelling at the child will only escalate the problem, as will losing your own temper, hitting, or even shouting insults.

So you tune into another force, which I think is love. You access your empathy and compassion for the child, and you recognize how much the child is suffering within her anger, perhaps even more than you are. You may need to respond with firmness, to set limits, to isolate the child or remind her of what might happen if the tantrum doesn't end. ("I can't bring you to the grocery store next time if you don't settle down right now.") But you respond from a place of love, not anger—which allows the child's anger to subside.

If you are an Anger type, you can engage in no better healing than to offer the people who upset you the same loving, firm response that a good parent might offer an angry child. I'm not suggesting that you become a patsy, that you allow others to walk all over you, submit blindly to aggression, or stop asking for what you need. I am suggesting that you try to view your "attackers" or "opponents" as small, angry children who are suffering in their tantrums, and that you rise to the level of a loving parent in your firm but compassionate response.

This is not an easy road to take. I have certainly found it challenging in both my therapy practice and my daily life. When someone treats you aggressively, insulting you or denying you your rightful due, it's very difficult not to respond with equal aggression, to try to force the other person to give you what you deserve, to insist that others acknowledge the rightness of your claims and the wrongness of their own actions.

Unfortunately, meeting aggression with greater aggression simply doesn't work. There are only three possibilities: Either you end up in a hostile confrontation that never ends, you lose the battle and feel worse than you did before, or you win the battle—and make a bitter enemy who is resolved to return one day and make you pay. In none of these situations are you truly acknowledged and appreciated. Even when you've won, you don't hear the sincere apology that your heart longed for, or receive the genuine appreciation that your soul required. And when you lose, you feel all the more humiliated for having fought so hard. The best you can hope for is a frustrating stalemate, a bitter loss, or a hollow victory.

If instead you are able to greet anger with love—a response that often requires tremendous discipline, practice, and inner strength—you'll be amazed at the positive results you reap. In the best-case scenario, your love will help to dissolve your "opponent's" aggression, just as a parent's firm calmness with a child can help to dispel a tantrum. Even if your opponent continues behaving with anger and resentment, you will walk away from the situation feeling better about yourself.

Anger locks us into endless battles that we will never win—battles that only make us feel worse about ourselves. Love, by contrast, frees us both from our own anger and from the anger of others, reminding us that we can always access our own larger selves and the joy they bring. This is a great offering that all of us can make to the world, to meet anger or aggression with calmness, firmness, and compassion, to see beneath the surface of another human being to what remains good and alive and hopeful in them. I don't find this easy, either in my therapy practice or in my daily life—but I do consider it one of the sacred vows that give meaning to the spiritual path of any tradition. And I know that this compassion is the only true antidote for the misery of being ruled by anger.

SELF-ACCEPTANCE AS THE KEY TO HEALING

Before I met him, Rick had already undergone long periods of traditional psychotherapy. But becoming more aware of his shortcomings without knowing how to "fix them" only made Rick feel worse. By the time I met him, Rick felt like someone lost deep in the woods with no one to guide him and no hope of ever getting out.

What I offered was another type of therapy, the Psychology of Mindfulness. This approach is based on great faith—the faith that inside each of us is everything we need to find freedom from our suffering; that there is more right than wrong within each of us; that as long as we are breathing, we have time to access our larger self and live in a world of joy (even if our pain never fully goes away).

Rick didn't need a therapist who could help him "fix" his life. He needed help learning to quiet his mind enough so that he could safely approach the mountain of anger that stood between him and his happiness. Once he could look at that mountain calmly, he could understand its place in his life and make different choices about how to respond to it. He needed to explore the terrain of his inner life and see what it was waiting to teach him. He needed to fully accept himself, his smallness as well as his largeness, his anger, blame, resentment, and rejection as much as his love, tenderness, and much-ignored capacity for compassion.

In fact, after Rick and I had created a space where Rick felt safe with his anger, it began to dissipate. He softened, and in our brief times together, his anger was set aside. Then we could begin working toward *awareness*, the first step toward mindfulness. Rick's anger had dominated his emotional landscape, like a bright flash of light that crowds out all other colors. He had to become aware of more subtle physical sensations—hurt feelings, for example, or bewilderment, or longing, or his own tenderness.

Rick also had to learn that by continually expressing and focusing on his anger, venting and attacking at the least provocation, he only made himself angrier. He had to learn to watch his language, to see that expressing his disappointment, over and over again, only gave it more solidity. Rick had to bring awareness to his speech, his behavior, even his thoughts, so that he could see how he was feeding his anger.

Gradually, Rick began to realize that the current source of his anger was himself. True, his friend's abuse and his parents' neglect were the embers that had long ago begun to burn within him. But now he was nourishing and stoking the flames by revisiting these memories time and again, and by finding new evidence for his victimhood in the present. Rick slowly saw that he had chosen to carefully tend the fires of his anger so that they never went out.

"Without my anger," he said one day, "I'll really have nothing.

They'll have done all those things to me—and I won't even have minded. My anger is the one thing about me that stands up for who I am."

Eventually, Rick became more aware of himself and less frightened of his own anger. Using the body awareness techniques in Chapter 15 helped him tune in to the other emotions he felt, besides anger: fear, sorrow, tenderness, sometimes even joy. He learned that his emotions were always changing, like sunlight flickering over water, and that he could calm himself through the Calming Breath Technique I described in Chapter 6. Gradually, he became able to enter into the furnace of his anger, to learn what it had to teach him.

Rick discovered that he, like most of us, had continued in his unhealthy pattern partly because he had always been unable to stop and look within. "It felt good to be angry," he told me after several months. Like so many people, Rick had gotten satisfaction from stoking the fires of justified anger, holding on to lifelong resentments, seeking to exact revenge on an uncaring world for what had been done to him. "But now I see," he concluded, "that I wasn't just hurting other people with my outbursts. I felt good at the time, but lousy afterward, like a drunk who never quite connects the hangover with the shot of bourbon. It *did* feel good to be angry—but in the end, it wasn't worth it."

RELEASING OUR EMOTIONS

Over time, Rick began to realize that his emotions were created first by thought. If he thought that the driver who cut him off in traffic was simply being a jerk, he'd get angry. But if he imagined that the very same driver was rushing to take a sick child to the hospital, he'd be understanding and would even pull back to make way. In both cases, the incident was the same—being cut off in traffic. But Rick's thoughts about the incident—"That's so unfair!" versus "I understand"—made the difference between an angry response and a compassionate one.

Emotions, Rick realized, are thoughts taking physical form, residing in the body. Their natural pattern is to flow, to move through the body like a stream or to rise and fall like a wave. It is when they become stagnant and stuck that they cause all kinds of problems. If, for example, Rick felt a momentary flash of anger as another driver cut him off, no harm done. The anger would pass in an instant, and Rick could return to his peaceful state. The problem came when the anger lingered on for minutes or even hours as Rick stoked its flames with further angry thoughts: "That jerk! Who does he think he is? How dare he cut me off? Doesn't he realize how dangerous that was? Besides, I'm in a hurry, too. That's the way accidents happen. . . ." Instead of signaling a problem and then passing quickly, the anger stagnated within Rick's heart, causing him far more pain than the momentary discomfort of the other driver's rudeness.

I sometimes see stuck emotions as debris that is clogging a mountain stream. As the debris accumulates, water backs up behind it. The pile of twigs and dead leaves begins to catch other floating pieces of debris, creating an ever-growing mountain of garbage that keeps the water from flowing.

Sometimes long-term psychotherapy can be like picking at the debris one piece at a time. It makes a difference, to be sure, but if the blockage is large, removing it piecemeal can feel like a hopeless task, especially since more junk is always floating downstream, adding to the blockage. Applying the understanding of mindfulness, by contrast, is like raising the level of water in the stream so that the debris is lifted up and easily carried away. Once the water is flowing, you can shift your awareness upstream and attend to the source of the debris. But you can experience the peace of a swiftly flowing steam even before you've fully understood what's wrong.

Thus, over time, Rick got better at distinguishing one feeling from another. Simply learning to distinguish between anger, fear, and sadness gave him some freedom from the tyranny of anger. He became more comfortable with his other feelings, willing to feel scared and lonely instead of channeling his discomfort into an ever-present rage. He also became more willing to let his emotions flow, to accept that his sadness or fear would not last forever.

OVERCOMING ANGER THROUGH COMPASSION

With time, Rick began to feel much better. He made a few friendships. He was able to repair some of his family relationships and let go of others. He was more content with his current job, but also aware of his desire for something better, and he was able to hold both of these thoughts with a sense of compassion for himself and hope for his future. He still had to do the inner work of finding and removing the source of the debris, the wound he had carried from childhood. But he could now do it from a place of strength and acceptance—including self-acceptance—rather than from a position of dominance and blame.

When the mind calms down, then the heart can open, which is what is was meant to do. Rick helped open his heart with a variation I created for him of the loving-kindness meditation described in Chapter 15. This exercise helped Rick stand firm in his newfound awareness and openheartedness so that he could go back in time and witness the events of his childhood, feeling compassion for his younger self and reaching out to comfort the vulnerable nine-year-old boy he had once been. He himself became the protective, soothing, loving presence that he had so longed for as a frightened child. Finally, Rick was healing himself.

For complete healing to occur, Rick had to move beyond himself to heal any ruptured relationships—in his case, his abuser and his parents, who hadn't known that they needed to stop the abuse. Rick is still working on forgiveness, in a process that may never be complete. Meanwhile, though, his life is opening up in ways that he wouldn't have considered possible even a few months ago. Most important, he's cultivating the capacity for love and his deepest longings are beginning to be fulfilled—not by the world giving him what he thinks he wants, but by his own transformation into a loving, compassionate man. Rick was learning that even the most difficult events can become a blessing if they force us to take a deep and reflective look inside.

"How will I know when my heart is healed?" Rick asked me once.

"The heart is healed when we express kindness," I replied. Rick liked this answer, because he understood that he could express kindness at any moment, even before his healing seemed complete. Every expression of kindness was both a cause and an effect of healing, in a process that would never end. I went on to share with him a statement that I'd once heard and never forgotten: "Life is so hard, how can we be anything but kind?"

14

SELF-DELUDING OR ADRIFT TYPES:
TRYING TO WAKE UP

"Are you a god?" they asked the Buddha.

"No," the Buddha replied.

"Are you an angel?"

"No," he replied again.

"Well, are you a saint?"

"No."

"Then what are you?"

"I am awake," the Buddha replied.

—TRADITIONAL BUDDHIST TALE

Lisa was a twenty-eight-year-old graduate student who had been with her current therapist for two years. She'd just come back from a school break in the midst of a crisis, and her therapist had never seen her so depressed. Although Lisa wasn't suicidal, she felt heavy and numb, her energy was very low, and she had lost virtually all interest and motivation. As a graduate student, she was particularly concerned about not being able to think clearly, which was causing her to fall behind in her schoolwork.

"Yes," Lisa told me, her tone flat, almost bored. "This is how I usually feel when I'm depressed." I could sense a deep sorrow, and a kind of distant anger buried within Lisa, but the face she presented to me was blank. "I usually shut down when things get overwhelming," she went on, and I marveled at how someone could speak so articulately and yet so neutrally about her own emotional state.

"I can get pretty spacey, and then I just need to sleep a lot," she explained. "I can't follow my normal routines, and sometimes it seems that I can't even think." When Lisa was depressed, she withdrew from the people in her life as well. She had trouble making even the simplest decisions—it had been difficult even for her to settle on a time for our appointment. "Basically, my life just grinds to a halt," she concluded.

THE FALSE SELF OF ABSENCE

As we've seen in previous chapters, we all have our favorite "false selves," or the small selves into which we withdraw when we're under stress. Denial types become confused, blank, numb and passive. It's almost as though they are trying to sleep through their lives, for fear of what might happen to them—what they might feel, or be called upon to do—should they be fully awake.

In Western terms, Lisa's pattern of symptoms is fairly typical of a classic form of depression previously known as melancholia or "involutional depression." On a chemical level, it's the result of insufficient norepinephrine and dopamine, the chemicals used to stimulate our brains. With depleted reserves of these crucial neurotransmitters, we find it difficult to remain awake, alert, and stimulated. As a result, we fall into the condition that fits the stereotyped view of depression: so tired and weighed down that it's literally difficult to get out of bed.

The classic Buddhist psychological term for this response is "delusional" which in Western psychiatry suggests psychosis and other problems that have nothing to do with the Buddhist definition. What the Buddhists are trying to get at, though, is the sense that this type breaks contact—almost deliberately—with some essential aspect of reality. Because something about reality seems too painful or overwhelming to deal with, the Denial type simply chooses to ignore it, to purposely—though unconsciously—block it out.

Like all of the unwise strategies we've considered, denial—setting oneself adrift—is an attempt to protect the small self. If a man is unhappy in his marriage, for example, and unable to imagine the consequences of confronting his spouse or setting in motion the process of divorce, he may choose to protect that fearful self by numbing out, refusing to feel the anger and sorrow at the injured marriage and avoiding the need to take some kind of action to either end or repair it. Likewise, if a woman is overwhelmed with obligations that she feels unable to refuse, she may become a kind of automaton, forcing herself through the daily round of joyless activities making herself numb so that she won't have to confront how burdened and resentful she feels. As with grasping and rejecting, setting oneself adrift comes at a tremendous cost, diminishing the self it was supposed to protect.

THE COSTS OF SHUTTING DOWN

Thus, Lisa was paying a huge price for her depression, which was interfering not only with her ability to take pleasure in her life, but also sabotaging her graduate-school career. What was unusual, she told me, was how suddenly her depression had come on. Although she'd felt this low before—several times—she'd never gotten to such a miserable place so quickly.

I asked Lisa if anything had triggered this crisis, and she said that she wasn't aware of anything. I wasn't surprised. It's typical of Denial types to be out of touch with their emotions just at the time when those emotions are most intense. Instead of recalling a painful incident with the anxiety, shame, or resentment that a Fear or Anger type might invoke, Lisa simply felt numb.

Since I was so certain that there had been a trigger, I probed further. Why, after two years of stability, had her depression returned? Was it seasonal? Menstrual? Had she changed her medication, her diet, her exercise habits, or her sleep cycles? Was she undergoing any relationship tensions—with a boyfriend, family member, or teacher?

No, Lisa kept repeating. Everything was going well.

"What about your break?" I asked. "What did you do with your time off?"

Lisa told me that she had traveled to visit a friend out of state, her best friend from college. "We had a great time," she insisted. "Margie just had a baby boy, and he was so cute. I love babies, and Margie let me feed him and bathe him and everything. She was so happy to be a mom—it was great to see the two of them together."

Still, I pointed out, her depression had started on this trip. Had there been any other point when she noticed her symptoms getting worse?

Yes, Lisa admitted, her mood had dropped when she'd gone to see a play at a local theater just a few days after she'd gotten back from visiting Margie. The show featured a poignant scene in which the main character expressed her grief over the death of her baby.

Suddenly Lisa began to cry, her flat, neutral tone dissolving in a stream of tears. "I wasn't really all that happy for Margie," she confessed. "I wanted to be, but I wasn't."

Lisa went on to tell me that she herself had had an abortion when she was just sixteen years old. In fact, shortly after that she'd become suicidal and was hospitalized. "But it can't be that," she insisted, wiping away the tears with the back of her hand. "I went over all that in therapy years ago."

Maybe she had talked about her abortion, I suggested. But her depression, and her tears, suggested that she had not fully grieved it. For over a decade now, Lisa had been carrying an extra burden of unresolved grief. Certainly, at age sixteen, Lisa wasn't equipped to handle the grief that she felt. So she did what many of us would do in those circumstances—she shut down. First, she got depressed. Then she tried to "get on with her life," "put all the pain behind her." But because her grief had never been felt and then released, it had gone underground.

Thus Denial types seem to carry a double burden. Not only are they upset, but they have no idea that they are upset. Lisa knew she was depressed, of course, but she denied for quite a while that there was any "reason" for it, any sorrow or anger behind the sluggishness and mental confusion. Her strategies of shutting down and withdrawing seemed to protect her, but they also incapacitated her from taking action.

Moreover, Lisa's behaviors were particularly painful for those who loved her—her roommate, her sister, and her boyfriend. They all had the sense that a part of Lisa was missing, that she was just going through the motions when they spent time together. I've had many clients whose mother or father was a Denial type, and they've spoken eloquently about how hard it is to have a parent who seems to be present but is in fact emotionally absent. Spouses, too, suffer from the absence of their partner, particularly when the partner continues to insist that nothing is wrong. As with all types of depression, the cost is paid not only by the people who shut down, but also by every person who cares about them.

THE PSYCHOLOGY OF ABSENCE

Like the other unwise strategies, the shutting down and "stuffing away" of Denial types is ultimately caused by fear: fear of what is or of what might be. Like all of us, Denial types fear conflict, suffering, and making a choice that doesn't turn out well. So when other strategies—wise or unwise—don't seem to work or don't come naturally to us, *denial* seems like an attractive alternative.

Although Denial types may use this tactic more readily than the rest of us, I don't believe there's a single human on earth who hasn't employed this "small self" strategy. Even the Buddha himself, before he accepted his true nature, was guilty of denial, while the biblical accounts of Moses and Jesus include episodes in which each of these religious figures refused to recognize their true nature until God finally forced them to do so. Denial is *the* default mechanism, the one that's always available even when others fail. It's like a fog always waiting to descend whenever we feel the need to obscure the painful reality before us. Like a narcotic, denial temporarily dulls our pain, although it certainly doesn't address our pain's root causes or eliminate it permanently. When the denial wears off, our pain is still there, as Lisa was discovering to her sorrow.

Even when the Fear or Anger types are guilty of denial, they usually have abundant—if incorrect—theories about why they're unhappy. They blame themselves, others, or life itself, but they insist that they know what's wrong. The Self-Deluding type, by contrast, usually has no idea. "You tell me," is one of their favorite phrases. "What do *you* think, doctor?" Lisa asked me, not once but several times. "What's my problem? What do I need?" Like most Denial types, hers was not a "what-if" mind or a "judging mind" but rather a "confused mind," a mind that was either unable or unwilling to face reality.

THE EPIDEMIC OF MINDLESSNESS

Fear types fit with the part of our culture that has often been called "the Age of Anxiety," while Anger types play out the pervasive aggression that marks both U.S. society and the world as a whole. It remains to Denial types to exemplify what I've come to call "the Culture of Mindlessness." While I'm not convinced that life is more stressful now than in times past, I am fairly certain that it is more hectic and distracted than at any other time in history. If you don't want to see things clearly, you've got innumerable distractions at your disposal, starting with the 24/7 work habits that so many of us are encouraged to adopt. If your cell phone is always on for that all-important call, if you're constantly checking your e-mail or working long hours from home, when do you have time to pause, reflect, and get in touch with your emotions? Even if you're not overwhelmed with work, you've got plenty of inducement to cloud your mind with pleasure—TV, video and computer games, home entertainment systems, and numerous other isolating entertainments are available, not to mention "mindless" social distractions like movies, sports events, and the crowded, noisy bar culture.

Of course any of these activities can be meaningful, inspiring, or at least relaxing. But it seems to be far easier to stay continually busy than it is to make time for solitude, contemplation, and silence. If you are part of U.S. culture and you'd rather be awake than asleep, you'd better make a deliberate, conscious choice, or it isn't likely to happen.

Slowing down is one way to stay awake. Breaking through denial is another. Of course it hurts to strip away the protective layers of denial and face the pain beneath. And beyond our individual denial of personal pain, we also suffer from a collective denial that allows problems to go on possibly to the point of no return. The major issues of our time—racism, poverty, hunger, war, environmental degradation, terrorism—are all prolonged by our collective unwillingness to see them clearly and our consequent inability to deal with them decisively. It seems to me that anyone who insists on bringing these "unacceptable" issues to our society's attention often faces the rage and pain of the collective denial that tries to blur or block out the problem.

The fear that causes an individual to shut down does more than prolong that person's pain—it also hurts the world at large. So long as the fog remains, it will prevent them from seeing things clearly, from finding his or her own voice, from responding to the reality that so urgently demands a response. Today, more than ever, we need people to live authentically, to find their voice and then speak loudly and clearly, to stand up for what is true and not be cowed by fear. We need people with courage. And courage begins where denial ends.

ENTERING THE CLOUD OF UNKNOWING

There is a classic book on Christian spirituality called *The Cloud of Unknowing*. Written hundreds of years ago by an anonymous Christian mystic, it describes with remarkable clarity the experience of being cut off from a relationship with the divine and the fullness of life. This cloud, wrote the medieval author, separates us from our selves and from the true experience of life that is really our birthright.

What creates this cloud? We do—by the way we perceive ourselves and the world. That deadness Lisa felt inside was the direct result of her own decision to turn off her attention. Just as Joe began to see lack everywhere and Rick started to resent everything, Lisa had become dead to all her experiences, all her perceptions blurred and obscured, as if she were barely able to open her sleepy eyes.

Certainly, I, too, have done my share of grasping, resenting, and "falling asleep." But for Lisa to wake up, she needed to understand that her inner deadness was a choice—albeit an unconscious one—to avoid suffering.

Lisa agreed that it would be more useful to recall the painful time of her abortion rather than to increase her medication. Although she knew having the abortion had been the right decision for her, she'd never had the chance to grieve over what it had meant. At the time, she'd been entirely focused on the practical side of things. Her complex mix of anger, guilt, shame, and loss seemed too much to deal with, particularly since she saw no clear path through this experience, no ritual to guide her, no family and friends gathering around to support her. She saw her pregnancy as her mistake, and she viewed the abortion as her choice. What place did grief have in all that?

I asked Lisa if she had any idea what to do *now* with all of these feelings. She did not. I asked if she would like to consider a mindfulness exercise that I had devised. "It's okay to feel the pain," I told her as she prepared to begin. "Don't be scared of it. Don't shut down in response to it. Let it in, and let it cleanse you. If your feelings aren't allowed to flow, they can reside in your body, where they stagnate and cause problems—physical, emotional, spiritual, or all three."

Then I talked Lisa through the following exercise. If you are trying to wake up from your denial or come to terms with a painful experience or simply see beneath the surface of your depression, you might try it, too.

Letting Your Feelings Flow
- Find a time in the next few days when your energy is fairly good and you won't be interrupted for an hour or so. Then sit quietly and direct your awareness to the heart center, or wherever else in the body that your attention feels drawn.
- Next, invite images to arise about the painful experiences. Know that you can handle these feelings, and that you may experience healing within a brief time, even in that moment. Let the memories be as vivid as possible, inviting feelings to arise.

- Notice any physical sensations. Where in your body do they reside? What is the emotion connected with that physical experience? Become aware of it, let it grow, and allow yourself to become very clear about it and what is behind it. Be curious and unafraid. As you observe it, does it move? Is it associated with pain or discomfort?

- If the experience is a painful one, just continue to observe, holding your awareness lightly on the pain. Try not to interrupt or close down in response to an unpleasant feeling. Just sit with it and experience it for as long as you can, as long as it feels alive and draws your attention.

- When you are ready, open your eyes and begin writing about the experience. Pour out everything there is to say at that moment, onto the paper. Think of yourself as drawing the experience out of your body and mind, and storing it on the page. Be conscious of your intention to let go of the buried feeling.

- Close with a ritual that symbolizes your releasing this long-held emotion. For example, you might begin the exercise by lighting a candle and end by blowing the candle out. Or you might wash your hands, slowly and lovingly, feeling yourself wash away the emotion you've released. You might engage in a few minutes of conscious breathing, feeling yourself release the emotion with every breath you exhale. Find a "releasing ritual" that feels right for you.

COMING AWAKE

Lisa returned two weeks later and talked about doing the exercise, which she found difficult but helpful. While she wasn't depression-free, the intensity of her suffering had eased. "The edge is gone," she told me, sounding a bit more lively. Although she knew she could always increase her medication if she needed to, she thought she was all right for now.

We both knew that Lisa had more work to do with these feelings and that her depression could always come back. Yet both Lisa and I could sense that she had somehow changed—subtly, but unmistakably. As I saw it, her eyes had been opened. Lisa now had some clarity about what was going on inside her, and how her current state had been influenced by events both current and remote. She also had begun to face the consequences of her early choices, and she'd seen that as she did so, the fog began to lift. While she did not yet feel happy, Lisa was beginning to feel alive. Although I wished her joy, I knew this was not yet her time for that. This was her time for tenderness.

Sometimes, we're simply brought to our knees—by depression, illness, a terrible loss, or some other circumstance that simply feels bigger than we are. The only way we can respond is to look up and look within. We all feel helpless at times—and sometimes accepting our helplessness is actually a way of being drawn toward our "salvation"— toward the healing insight or experience that literally "salves," nurtures, heals, creates. Think of Kisa Gotami, the woman who lost her child— and found a whole new approach to life. Or think of great works of art, literature, and spirituality. Many are born out of a brush with despair.

I once knew a real-life Kisa Gotami, a man who lost a child who was very dear to him. I marveled at the wisdom he seemed to find as he came awake to his own life in a whole new way—torn almost violently awake by the grief and loss he had suffered. When I commented on this one day, he smiled ruefully and said, "Yeah, if I had the choice, I'd be stupid, and have my daughter back. But since I had no choice, I accepted the wisdom."

Lisa, too, might have wished for the choice to rewrite her life without the painful event that had set her on the path to depression. But as she slowly awakened, she made the best of the choice she actually had. She began to find a way to transform her greatest sorrow into her greatest joy, not by erasing the sorrow, but by making room for the joy alongside it. The pain that led her to "put herself to sleep" became the painful, joyous occasion of her new awakening.

STRATEGIES OF WISDOM

Mindfulness is our primary tool for staying awake. It sounds so simple. All you have to do is remain aware. Well, it may not be easy, but it *is* simple. You only have to be present in every moment. But there are so many things that do take us out of the moment, and the force of their pull is strong. The next chapter will offer you some specific strategies for becoming mindful, for waking up your mind, heart, and soul. Here, I'll share with you the major qualities you'll need to feed in order to become truly mindful.

- **Acceptance.** The Jesuit teacher and scholar Anthony De Mello wrote something in his book *Awareness* that I've never forgotten. He said that one of the most important messages in every religious tradition was the simple statement "All is well."

If we can fully embrace the truth of that statement—if we can accept that on the deepest possible level, everything is as it should be—then we truly have nothing to fear. It is safe to open our eyes and hearts. It is safe to come out and play. It is safe to wake up to our lives.

Acceptance does not mean seeing the world through rose-colored glasses. That would be just another form of denial. Rather, acceptance means seeing things as clearly as we can, no matter what then seems to be required of us. If denial leads to passive resignation—the numb acquiescence of a bad marriage, the fearful agreement to an unfair boss—acceptance means a wholehearted understanding of the truth of our lives, our feelings, and our world. If this understanding then requires us to act against injustice or to confront a painful situation, so be it. Leaving an abusive spouse, challenging an alcoholic coworker, giving voice to our political frustrations, stepping in to halt an environmental debacle—these are only some of the responses we may feel compelled to make once we have become fully aware and accepting of the reality within which we live.

- **Courage.** If awareness and acceptance are required of the mind, then courage is what is required of the heart. Fearless awareness allows us to face whatever is before us, both a prerequisite and a result of living with our eyes wide open. We need a bit of courage—or at least faith—to open our eyes in the first place. But each time we see things as they really are and then take the action we believe is required, we reinforce and expand our store of courage.

Most people are committed to staying in illusion, a comfortable dream state that permits them to remain passive. It's what they know—it's what everyone seems to know, and so it seems right and normal. It takes tremendous courage, faith, and persistence to insist that the emperor has no clothes, to refuse to follow false gods, to speak and act from a place of truth and clarity.

Like every positive quality of the heart, courage can be cultivated. First, it is planted with the seeds of intention. Then it is watered with mindful acceptance. It is cultivated by practices of the heart. And finally, it is harvested. If you would like to "grow" your courage, approach Chapter 15 with this intention. And never make the mistake of believing that you don't have the courage you need for an act you believe is right. If you don't have the courage, you can find it or create it. Courage, like all other qualities, is a process, not a fixed commodity. By invoking it, you bring it to life.

- **Presence.** What are the fruits of that harvest of courage? How can we see and know the person who is awake?

  When a person is awake, he is truly present in the moment. She is full of vitality, responsive and alive.

  An awake person is fully embodied. That is, he resides completely in his body. He is not estranged from it; he doesn't ignore it. He has learned to listen to his body, to honor it. He accepts his body as it is, knowing that it needn't be perfect in order for him to befriend it. He is attuned to his body, knowing what it needs and seeking to provide it.

  An awake person is also aware. Her mind is quiet yet alert, ready to go to work when called upon but willing to stay in the background when the thinking mind is not required. She observes herself and all that is before her, unafraid, not needing to cling to any part of reality nor to push it away, simply allowing it to be as it is. She can then decide whether to take action and choose the action that seems most effective.

  An awake person has a heart that is open and engaged. He no longer feels a need to close his heart or shrink away to protect himself. When a feeling arises, he is aware of it and welcomes it. He neither suppresses his negative emotions nor fans them, for he knows that both reactions only keep such feelings alive. Instead, he allows every negative emotion to rise within him, have its life, and then pass away.

  An awake person has tended to her mind and heart, and has consciously chosen the path of wisdom. She has created within herself the capacities for generosity, compassion, forgiveness, courage, love.

  Engaged, yet detached. Active, yet calm. Moving, yet still. *This* is how it is to be awake in the world. Your goal is to be awake. The world is very good at hypnosis, at dulling your consciousness. But you want to be more alive, more fully embodied in this life.

  Seeing all that is, you recognize that life is full of good things. Think of them now, think of them often. Fill your heart with gratitude and you will be both happy *and* awake. If you are awake to the blessings that life offers, you are truly awake.

15

STRATEGIES OF WISDOM

Research is just beginning to be done on the long-term effectiveness of mindfulness in promoting both physical and mental health. But as a longtime practitioner, both in my own life and as a teacher, workshop leader, and psychotherapist, I can attest to the near-miraculous effects of mindfulness practice. If you set aside as little as five minutes a day, five days a week, to devote to some of the exercises in this chapter, you'll begin to notice that you're calmer, more open, less stressed. You may notice that you're sleeping better, getting along better with loved ones and colleagues, and feeling more hopeful. You may also learn more about yourself, discover hitherto unsuspected dreams and desires, or develop a new relationship to your spiritual life.

I personally would recommend a mindfulness practice that includes at least twenty to thirty minutes a day, five days a week. It may be helpful to do even more during those times when you are facing particularly severe stress. But mindfulness practice should not become another source of guilt, shame, or self-blame! Do what you can, as you can do it, and let your practice take its own course. Read through this chapter and let your intuition be your guide as to which exercises will be most meaningful or helpful for you.

WHAT IS MINDFULNESS?

When defining mindfulness, I like to rely on the definition I learned from Jon Kabat-Zinn when I first studied with him fifteen years ago:

"Mindfulness is awareness, from moment to moment, on purpose, without judgment."

Awareness is another word for the condition of being awake. As I said in Chapter 14, being awake means being "Engaged, yet detached. Active, yet calm. Moving, yet still." *Purpose* is another word for "intention," the quality of choosing and acting consciously, rather than reacting automatically. And being without judgment requires us to expand our capacity for acceptance—both self-acceptance and acceptance of others.

I recently read a lovely story about acceptance in the works of Islamic philosopher Idries Shah. Like many ancient teaching stories, this one involves a wise fool, sort of a sacred clown, who manages to fumble his way into wisdom—Mullah Nasrudin, the foil for many Islamic tales.

In this story, Mullah Nasrudin has taken up gardening. He loves the flowers and vegetables that he grows, and he becomes an adept gardener. But his garden is plagued by dandelions, and Nasrudin begins to grow more and more frustrated at his inability to control them.

Finally, Nasrudin can bear the dandelion invasion no longer. He travels to the city to consult the Prince's gardener, acknowledged throughout the land for his mastery of gardening, and begs for help. The royal gardener gives Nasrudin instructions for the most effective remedy he knows.

Mullah Nasrudin goes home, full of enthusiasm, and follows the royal gardener's instructions to the letter. But still, the dandelions return, just as they always have.

Really angry now, Nasrudin goes back to the master gardener. "You're a fraud!" he declares. "Your remedy was no better than the rest! What else can I do about these dandelions?"

The master gardener looks thoughtful and strokes his chin. Finally, he says softly, "Mullah Nasrudin, there is only one thing to do. You must learn to love the dandelions."

In a similar way, mindfulness practice suggests that we give up on self-improvement and instead begin a course of self-acceptance. The way out of our unhappiness is not to fix ourselves. We can't root out our flaws any more than Nasrudin can destroy every single one of his dandelions. We might try for years, and the dandelions would still remain.

There is only one thing to do. We must learn to love the dandelions.

STAYING WITH OUR OBSERVING SELF

Imagine that you are sitting beside a stream, comfortably situated on the bank. You are completely calm and at ease, awake and alert. As you sit there, you notice something floating in the stream—a log, a piece of debris, perhaps a boat or something else that interests you. You remain still and continue to observe, as first one thing and then another passes by, some that interest you, some that do not. But however you feel, whatever you think about the items in the stream, you simply sit, noticing each object as it comes, letting it pass, and then turning your attention to the next object that comes along.

This is what it is like to align yourself with the observing self. Although it notices everything that passes by on the stream of your consciousness, it remains coolly unaffected. Your thoughts proceed, one after another, some dull and routine, others more interesting and unusual.

Sometimes, a really dramatic or compelling thought may come along. When that happens, your small self is so attracted that it wants to jump into the water. Sometimes your small self thrashes about, agitating the previously calm surface of the stream. Other times it tries to hold on to the object, refusing to let it pass farther downstream. "This is the most important object in the world," thinks your small self. "This is reality! I don't want to let go."

But the larger observing self just stays on the bank and calmly takes it all in. It does not judge what comes by as good or bad but recognizes each thought as something that is produced by your mind and does not represent the whole of reality. The observing self does not even judge the small self for getting so caught up in jumping into the stream. It understands that every item that comes along is only a thought, with no more power than we choose to give it.

What makes this practice so useful? When you observe this process, you begin to understand that the mind's job is simply to generate thoughts. Some are more useful than others, but none in themselves are either good or bad. But when you understand that the mind is only generating thoughts, then you can choose which thoughts to entertain, which to believe, and which to discard or let die.

Remember that mindfulness, like everything else, takes practice. Expecting it to work effortlessly, or overnight, is a recipe for disappointment. But sooner or later, you will begin to see the effects of your practice. And then, when you want to rely on your larger self to get you through a crisis, you'll know you can.

GET IN TOUCH WITH YOUR BREATH

A good place to begin meditation is by becoming aware of your breathing. Indeed, some advanced practitioners rely on conscious breathing as their primary form of practice. Your breath is always there, always moving, always reminding you that life is built upon cycles.

Awareness of Breathing
- Sit comfortably, with your back upright but not rigid.
- Close your eyes, or look gently at a place on the floor four to five feet in front of you.
- Place the tip of your tongue on your palate just behind and above your teeth.
- Breathe through your nose, if you can.
- Focus all your attention on each breath, with as much interest as if it were something you had never before experienced.
- Observe the movement of your belly up and down. Experience it as if you were riding upon gentle waves.
- You don't need to change your breath in any way—just observe it. Notice everything about your breathing: the movement of air in and out of your nose; your breath's temperature as it comes in and goes out; the flow of air into your chest; the expansion of your chest in all directions; the still point between inhale and exhale. Then notice the whole process in reverse.
- Do this exercise for five to ten minutes, once or twice daily. Each time you realize that you are no longer aware of your breath, gently release whatever thoughts absorbed you and return to a deep experience of your breathing.

OBSERVE THE MIND

Sitting meditation is intended to give you a lens into your inner life—to let yourself focus on the thoughts and feelings that flow through you. You don't undertake this process with any goal in mind; your only object is to have whatever experience comes up for you. You'll get the most from your meditation by grounding yourself in the notion that whatever happens is fine—no matter what occurs, you can observe it and learn from it.

People who've never meditated before often have preconceived ideas of what you "should" and "shouldn't" feel. I can testify from my own experience that sometimes you'll feel deeply relaxed, and other times you'll be so restless you wonder why anyone bothers with this annoying practice. Sometimes when I meditate, I feel real contentment; other times, I feel bored; still other times, I ache with the pain of difficult emotions, troubling memories, or just a diffuse grief that seems to have no source. Occasionally I'm visited by great ideas and unexpected insights.

No matter what comes up when I meditate, I try to simply observe without judging. I admit, I sometimes find it hard not to decide that contentment is good and pain is bad, to feel proud of having a serene and joyous experience when I meditate and ashamed of being restless. What I try to do, though—and what I counsel you to do—is simply to observe and learn. Think of yourself in the spirit of a scientist studying gorillas in the wild—filled with curiosity, wonder, and awe.

By the way, sitting meditation is a bit harder to learn than some of the other practices in this chapter, so I recommend you seek some guidance, especially early on. Many people are able to learn this technique by using a tape, but when I was first learning to meditate, I appreciated having someone to answer my questions, and I also found it helpful to hear about the experience of my fellow students. Look for a class in Mindfulness-Based Stress Reduction, the process developed by Jon Kabat-Zinn.

Sitting Meditation

- Sit comfortably, your back upright but not rigid. You may sit on a meditation cushion, bench, or chair. Try not to slouch or lean back in the chair. Imagine yourself sitting up straight (but relaxed), with your head erect and floating directly above your spine.
- Close your eyes, or look gently at a place on the floor four to five feet in front of you.
- Place the tip of your tongue on your palate, just behind and above your teeth.

- Breathe through your nose, if you can.
- Check your posture to make sure you're comfortable. If you need to shift your body at any point, go ahead, rather than letting discomfort interfere with your meditation.
- Begin with a few moments of Awareness of Breathing. Use your own breath as your touchstone. Return to it whenever you realize that your mind has wandered off, and stay with your breath until you've regained your conscious awareness.
- Expand your field of awareness to include your body and any sensations floating through it. You might notice again how you are sitting, remarking upon any discomfort you feel, or keying in to the feeling of your warm and heavy hands resting upon your legs. Allow anything in your body that calls to you to be the focus of your awareness.
- You can also become aware of outside sensations, like the movement of the air or any sounds around you. Instead of seeing these external events as a distraction, experience them as part of the moment. Anything in your world—anything at all—can be approached with openness and awareness.
- After a few moments of sensory awareness, expand your focus again to include the act of thinking. Hold in your mind the image of yourself sitting by the banks of a river as your observer self watches your thoughts arise, and then fall. As soon as one thought evaporates, another comes to take its place. Just sit and notice, trying not to let any thought carry you away and out of the moment.
- You can use anything as a moment of mindfulness: even your distraction and your sense that your awareness has weakened. Without blame or judgment, simply say to yourself, "Ah, I see that my mind has taken me away again." And again, and again, and again . . . It happens repeatedly to all of us. Just notice the experience, let it go, and return to your breath for a few cycles. Then focus on simply sitting and observing your thoughts.
- Practice sitting in this way for fifteen to forty-five minutes, as often as you can.

MEDITATE WITH MOVEMENT

Another way to engage the body in meditation is through Walking Meditation. Like the Awareness of Breathing Meditation, this is a favorite with both beginning and advanced practitioners of mindfulness. Because it involves movement, it's a nice option when one is sleepy or the mind is scattered. It may be particularly appealing for Air types, who like movement, or for Earth types who are trying to overcome sluggishness. You can use it as either an alternative or in addition to a more formal sitting meditation. You can also incorporate it into your daily activities, for just a few minutes or for up to an hour.

∽∾

Walking Meditation

- Try to do this meditation without focusing on a goal. Try walking just for the sake of being aware of walking, and not for exercise, seeing the sights, or getting somewhere.
- Begin by standing still with your feet about hip width apart. Try to distribute your weight evenly between both feet, and also between the heels and balls of your feet. Place your hands in front of you, waist high, palms up with one on top of the other and thumbs touching. Or place your hands behind you with your fingers laced together.
- Keep your eyes open, but with only a soft focus on the ground a few feet ahead.
- Start out very slowly, noticing how your weight shifts onto one foot as you raise the heel of your opposite foot off the ground. Pay attention to the bending of your knee, the way your whole foot comes off the ground, your leg rising and coming forward, your hip shifting, your knee extending as you prepare to plant your foot in front of you.
- Experience your heel coming onto the ground, followed by your mid- and forefoot. Feel how your toes stretch out and balance you. Notice how your weight now shifts onto this forward foot, and the way your other heel lifts gently off the ground as your weight shifts.
- Try to experience each aspect of your movement in minute detail, at least initially. Allow your attention to be drawn to your body as the movement continues.
- After a few minutes, when it feels as though you are really present in the experience, try moving a little faster. Vary your speed, always keeping your moment-to-moment experience foremost in your awareness.
- You don't need to go anywhere. You may simply want to walk back and

forth over a stretch of several yards. Again, your focus is on the experience of walking, and not what you see or where you go.

- As with any meditation, your mind will occasionally wander. As soon as you notice this loss of focus, just bring your awareness back to the present moment and to your experience of walking.

DWELLING IN THE HEART

Pema Chodrin is one of today's most beloved Buddhist teachers. She uses a lovely metaphor to describe the heart and the problems that occur when it is closed.

The heart, she says, is like a sea anemone, a small creature that plants itself on the ocean floor and feeds on nutrients in the water. Its mouth is an opening at the top that is very soft in the center, surrounded by numerous waving tentacles that help to draw food inward. But when the anemone feels threatened, it closes up tightly, pulling its softness inside for protection and presenting a tough exterior to the outside world.

The anemone, says Chodrin, is protected. But closed off and shut up tight, it can't access the nutrients in which it is bathed. If the anemone stays closed for too long, it will starve.

Closing down in the face of danger wouldn't present a problem if we opened up again as soon as the threat was gone. But many of us have closed down so often, or for such long periods of time, that we have forgotten how to open our hearts at all. Our innocent attempt to protect ourselves comes at a great personal cost. And if we stay closed down long enough, we may begin to believe that no food exists. Eventually, we, too, risk starving in a sea of plenty, when all we needed to nourish ourselves was to open our hearts.

One of the reasons that our hearts become heavy or closed is that we have trouble enduring the difficult emotions—fear, anger, or sadness. Although we are designed to experience a wide range of feelings—from joy to despair and everything in between—we often decide that we should always feel happy or satisfied. When these longed-for emotions don't arise, we slip automatically into our favorite strategy: grasping, pushing away, or shutting down. Then our reaction to any less-than-pleasant emotion makes us feel worse than the feeling itself.

How much happier we'd be if we could simply accept our emotions—the negative as well as the positive—without judging either ourselves or our lives when we "feel bad." The mystic poet Rumi invokes this idea in his poem "The Guest House," in which he says that the human condition is like a guesthouse, with each of us receiving visitors every day—emotions and insights. We should welcome them all, Rumi suggests, even "a crowd of sorrows," for they may be preparing us for something new, something greater. "Be grateful for whoever comes," Rumi concludes, "for each has been sent as a guide from beyond."

THE SOURCE OF EMOTION

I often tell my patients that emotions are actually thoughts translated into physical experience. Think about something sad, and you will likely feel sad. Your eyes may tear up, your heart feels heavy, and you being to feel slow and tender. Think about something maddening, and you'll probably feel anger as your breath quickens, your heart races, and, perhaps, your chest tightens. The more powerful your imagination, the better you are able to generate feelings with your mind. And the more you believe in what you're thinking, the more likely that your mind will turn your thoughts into an emotion.

When we're functioning as our healthy, resilient larger selves, our emotions can come and go like visitors, moving through our bodies but not taking up permanent residence. When we're stuck emotionally, struggling with low resilience, or committed to clinging to negative thoughts, our emotions may lodge in our organs, muscles, or bones, causing discomfort, pain, or even disease.

The irony is that we need all our emotions, the negative as well as the positive. If we can't experience our emotions, we don't know when we're being hurt and we can't take steps to solve a problem or move away from the people or situations that are hurting us. I often see people in unhealthy relationships or workplaces who don't act to help themselves because they're ignoring the signals that their emotions are sending them. Either they've become numb to their painful feelings, or they've never learned how to interpret or act upon them.

Feelings can also be our guide to our current state of mind. Having an unpleasant feeling can signal us that something is off in our thinking. If we find ourselves feeling anxious, envious, or numb, we can realize that we've fallen prey to faulty thoughts, which in turn have given rise to these emotions. Instead of investing in the negative feeling, we can treat it as a guide—a sort of warning light flashing on our dashboard, signaling us that we're low on gas or that our car's electrical wiring is malfunctioning. "I'm envious," we might think. "So there's something I'm missing about how full my life is, or how much I need to make some changes. I'm caught in a mistaken belief that someone else's happiness comes at my expense, or that there's not enough in the world for me, too."

Or, "I'm anxious. Why? I feel so alone and abandoned. I'm having the thought that my life will always be empty and friendless. But it's only a thought. I can't really *know* what the future will bring. My mind is drawing me into one frantic thought after another—and these thoughts are making me anxious. How can I correct those thoughts?"

Observing our feelings without judgment or blame frees us to correct our faulty thoughts and to seek perceptions that are truer. We can actually welcome our negative emotions—and then release them, rather than either suppressing our feelings or holding on to them.

NAVIGATING UNHEALTHY MOODS

What do we do when a negative emotion really takes hold, lingering over us like a damp, dark cloud? A "bad mood" of this type can be particularly frightening for anyone who has ever undergone depression, because you know that these moods can easily turn into full-blown depression.

The best thing you can do with a bad mood is to welcome it with awareness and acceptance. Reacting automatically with grasping, rejecting, or shutting down only serves to pull you further into the mood. Giving your mood too much attention—commiserating with a friend or ruminating about what's wrong—may only feed your bad feeling and give it more strength. Numbing out and trying to comfort yourself with addictive or unhealthy behaviors will also make your mood worse.

On the other hand, distracting yourself intentionally might help your mood to lift. Sometimes it helps just to occupy your mind with something else: a change of scenery, a funny movie, a friend who's healthy enough (at the moment, at least) that he or she won't support your negativity. Doing something purposely to break a bad mood is not denial. It's just good common sense.

If you wait patiently without feeding your bad mood, the mood may simply move on. Bringing mindful awareness to the situation can really help, because it gives you plenty of evidence that moods are constantly changing—that is simply their nature. Even in the midst of a hard time, you experience good feelings as well as bad, though many of us don't realize that this is so. Learning to become more observant, to notice the ever-changing play of sunlight and shadow on the stream of our consciousness, can help you remember that emotions come and go, freeing you from the grip of your bad mood and inspiring faith that you'll come out of it. That faith in turn loosens the grip of fear, anger, and confusion, making it even easier to move on.

RELEASING NEGATIVE EMOTIONS

Imagine that you are clutching a pen in your hand. How do you release it? You open your hand and let it go. But even with such a simple act, the process begins with your mind. First you create a thought, or an intention: "I will release this pen." Then your brain sends a signal to your hand to release the muscles of contraction that have been holding the pen. Once these muscles have released their grip, you need only a small amount of effort from your muscles of opening. Finally, you release the pen.

This is how your heart operates as well. When you become aware that you are holding on to some emotion that no longer serves you, you can decide consciously whether you are willing to release it. If you are, then you can create that intention in the mind and set the mechanics of release in motion. Most of the work is done just by ceasing to grip the emotion.

Of course most of us have more trouble letting go of unpleasant emotions than releasing a pen from our hand. For a time, you may repeatedly pick up an old emotion, perhaps out of habit or because you're not really ready to be done with it. But with a mindful approach, you'll soon realize what you're doing and can then choose how to respond.

Just as with the pen, you release a nonuseful emotion in a series of steps. First, you must realize that the negative feeling exists in your own heart. Becoming aware of your emotion is necessary—and surprisingly hard for many people, who bury their grief, anger, and fear so deep that they've stopped being conscious of all the weight they carry. So awareness, as always, is the first step.

Once you've noticed your troublesome feeling, you must "own" it. Often our self-image interferes with our ability to acknowledge the feeling we've identified. "I never get angry, it's just not worth it," a sweet-tempered woman might say. When her anger makes itself unmistakably known, she gets stuck in denying that someone like her could possibly feel such a thing. Or a man might insist that he's not really sad, just a little tired. Resentment, envy, greed, and fear are only some of the emotions that we often find difficult to acknowledge.

Next comes the realization that your feeling has served its purpose. You felt fearful of speaking in public because you once had such a fragile sense of self that you needed to protect yourself from every possible occasion for ridicule—but you're stronger than that now. You felt sad about a broken romance, but you're done with mourning and ready to move on. You felt angry about a perceived injustice—but you've responded to the best of your ability and must now let your anger go.

Having understood that you no longer need a particular emotion, you form an intention to release it, and—whether you do this immediately or take a while—you eventually become willing to let the feeling go. Finally, you take action to release the emotion that no longer serves you, making room for a new feeling to take its place.

Now imagine a man whose hand is so strongly contracted that anything he picks up has to be pried from his grip. Perhaps he's been clutching that particular pen too hard, or his hand has been contracted for so long with other things that it's forgotten how to release. The man may need another person to help him remove the pen. But with time, hopefully, he can be taught to relax his grip.

Sometimes our heart has constricted so strongly, or our emotions are so sticky, that we have trouble releasing our feelings. If your heart is too tightly closed, or if you don't know how to open it, you can work on cultivating what Buddhist psychologists call a "good"—that is, a loving—heart.

Working Through Emotional Blockages with Awareness
- Turn your awareness to the heart. Let yourself become aware of the feeling and of your willingness to let it go.
- Make the connection between a physical sensation in the body and a particular negative emotion. Learn to pinpoint the emotion to a spe-

cific location in the body, and to describe the physical feeling in words.

- Become aware of negative emotions as soon as they arise. Don't judge either yourself or your feeling as bad. Simply see it as a sign that you have been pulled off center—just for that moment. Use that awareness to bring you back into the moment.

- Accept your feeling completely. Don't feel the need to push it away or focus on wishing it were otherwise. When you accept a negative feeling, the negativity loses some of its hold on you.

- Knowing that you have created this feeling (however legitimately in response to your circumstances), realize that you are the only one who can release or "uncreate" the feeling.

- Bring your awareness to your breath. Then, if circumstances allow, focus directly on the negative emotion itself. Let yourself feel it fully, without fear. Notice all that you can about it—where it is in your body, how it feels, whether it moves or changes from moment to moment.

- Be honest with yourself as you assess whether you are ready to release this feeling or if you'd prefer to hold on to it a while longer.

- If you feel ready to let go, allow yourself to become aware of a sensation of movement, flow, or expansion, somewhere in your midsection (usually the heart center).

- With each inhale, let yourself be fully aware of the feeling, fully accepting of it. You may say to yourself: "As I breathe in, I feel————."

- With each exhale, invite the feeling to recede, to flow out of yourself. You may say, "As I breathe out, I release————."

- Invite your heart to open and the negative feeling to be released. See yourself let it go. Visualize it floating away, like a log on a river or a pen falling from your hand.

- Do this for as long and as often as needed. End with a ritual, like writing or a symbolic releasing.

Note: If it's unclear why you've created the feeling, why it won't leave, or why it keeps coming back, you may find it helpful to do a dialogue journal (discussed later in this chapter), or discuss it with someone trained in this approach.

Heart-Opening Meditation
- Sit quietly in a comfortable position.
- Focus upon several breaths, allowing your mind to settle.

- Bring your awareness to your heart center, the area in the middle of your chest, just below your breastbone. You can gently place your hand over this area.
- Notice whatever feeling arises in your heart center, setting aside all judgment or need for your feelings to be different than they are.
- Become aware of the degree of openness that you experience at this moment. When your heart is open, you will notice a sense of expansion, flowing, fullness, lightness, or warmth. When your heart is closed, it feels tight, stagnant, empty, heavy, or cool. Try not to judge one condition as good and the other bad. Just notice and accept whatever is true for you now, and know that your feelings are always changing.
- Now bring to mind a time in the recent past when you were moved by something that touched your heart—a kind word, a thoughtful act, a compliment, a caress, a surprise of beauty, a shared sorrow. Recall the experience as vividly as you can, including the other person(s) involved, the setting, and any associated smells, colors, or sounds. Experience, for as long as you like, the feeling that you had at the time.
- Invite your heart to open ever so slightly. Observe it. Experience the feeling that you have when it opens.
- If no specific image or memory came up for you, simply hold the intention to let the heart soften and open now, in this moment.
- End with total acceptance and gratitude for whatever your experience of this process has been.

CULTIVATE THE CONDITIONS FOR GENEROSITY

Think of someone you know who seems to be really happy. What's his or her relationship to giving and receiving? The happiest people I know are clearly generous. They seem able to give and receive with equal delight. They don't cling or try to keep things, people, or experiences for themselves. They get as much joy from seeing someone else do well as they do from having their own triumphs. They might as well be saying, "Your happiness is my happiness."

Working with the heart in the intentional way I'm describing in this chapter gives us a wonderful opportunity to create the kind of life that we truly want to have. Even if we start out not believing ourselves to be happy or generous, we accept that it's at least possible that we possess these good qualities and seek to become good by creating the conditions within ourselves that make it possible. With the mind, we can look at our beliefs about abundance. We can see it up close and personal, which gives us at least a fighting chance of changing it. Working with the heart, with even a sliver of an opening, we can go in and repeatedly plant the seeds of generosity. We can cultivate the feeling of gratitude, and we can endeavor to wish well for others.

You can engage in the following meditation for just a few minutes, or for an extended period of time. You can also incorporate it into your daily time for mindfulness meditation. However you engage in this meditation, do this often. I particularly recommend it for the close of the day, reflecting back on what you are grateful for from the day.

A Meditation on Gratitude
- Sit quietly in a comfortable position.
- Focus upon several breaths, allowing your mind to settle.
- Bring your awareness to your heart center.
- Notice whatever feeling is in your heart at this moment, and accept it just as it is.
- Maintaining some awareness of the heart, bring an image to mind of someone who has helped you or been kind to you, now or in the past. You may think of a teacher, a mentor, a friend, a loved one, or even a stranger.
- Allow the image of this person, and the good he or she has done for you, to become very clear.
- Imagine that the person is standing right before you. Invite him or her to come closer. Look the person in the eye, and give him or her your thanks.
- Try to be as specific as you can in saying what you are grateful for.
- Allow the image to fade, but spend a few more moments lingering with your awareness of gratitude.
- If you like, repeat the process with other people, things, or events for which you are grateful.
- You might want to write down what came up for you after the meditation.

ACT GENEROUSLY

Would you like to know the true secret of generosity? It's another one of those principles that seems so simple but can be so difficult to assimilate:

Giving and receiving are one and the same. Whatever you do for others, you also do for yourself. The best way to make yourself feel rich and full is to make a heartfelt gift to someone else.

"Never suppress a generous impulse," counseled the Greek philosopher Epictetus. Whenever you have the thought to give something away, do so. Our gifts might take a humble form—a smile, a touch, some of our time, our listening presence, assistance, money—but whatever they are, we can give generously, with gratitude that we have it to give in the first place. Today, as I was walking through an unfamiliar neighborhood in a nearby city, I encountered a homeless man who held out a cup for spare change. My arms were full of packages, and it had started to rain. I apologized that I wasn't able to give him anything, and he smiled at me.

"That's all right, man," he said with a genuine warmth that caught me off guard. "You better get on now—the rain's going to come down harder any minute."

I was so taken aback by his concern for me that I began to rearrange my packages so I could get at my wallet.

"It's okay, it's okay," he kept saying. "Just get out of the rain." When I described this encounter to a cynical friend, she insisted that the man's apparent concern for me was just a clever ploy to get me to give him more money. Perhaps she was right—but I don't think so. This homeless man had somehow retained an open, generous heart, and even in the midst of his suffering and need, he'd found a way to make himself feel rich.

⟆⟆⟆

Cultivating a Generous Heart
- Sit quietly in a comfortable position.
- Focus upon several breaths, allowing your mind to settle.
- Bring your awareness to your heart center.
- Notice whatever feeling is in your heart at this moment, and accept it just as it is.
- Bring to mind someone who is really happy and successful. With a clear image of this person, and as much generosity as you can muster, offer this person a phrase such as:
  - *May your happiness grow and be with you always.*

– *May your success continue.*

– *Your joy makes me happy.*

- You may continue this with others who have varying degrees of happiness.

- This practice can be done not just when meditating, but when you are out among people and noticing their joy or good fortune.

⁊ⱨⱨⱬ

EXPANDING OUR COMPASSION

If I had only one spiritual prescription to make for those of you suffering from depression, it would be to become more compassionate. Find new occasions to feel genuinely for the sorrow of another, and to express your compassion accordingly.

Now, why would I suggest that someone struggling with depression try to become more compassionate? At first glance, you might think people with depression are the ones who need compassion, not the other way around.

In fact, the effort to develop compassion involves precisely this shift in our identity. Are we someone who suffers or who relieves suffering? Are we a person who is driven by fear or someone who is moved by love? Encouraging ourselves to act with compassion is to embrace a vision of our larger selves, to understand that we are loving people who, despite our depression, can experience the essential human response of reaching out to care for those whom we see are suffering. Many obstacles can interfere with this natural response, primarily our own fear. So acting from a courageous, loving place reinforces our strength, our joy, our ability to celebrate life. Paradoxically, seeing the suffering life brings and then acting to relieve it is one of the most profound ways of saying yes to life.

The story is told that Gandhi was once approached by a man with a gun who intended to shoot him. But at the last minute, the assassin couldn't bring himself to commit the murder, and he was captured. As the man was being taken away, Gandhi is said to have remarked, "Oh my, what will happen to that man now?" That is an example of a heart that is free from fear—and full of compassion.

⟨⟫

A Meditation on Compassion

- Sit quietly in a comfortable position.
- Focus upon several breaths, allowing your mind to settle.
- Bring your awareness to your heart center.
- Notice whatever feeling is in your heart at this moment, and accept it just as it is.
- Bring to mind an image of yourself, now or in the past, when you needed kindness or comfort but did not receive it. Allow your feeling to change in response to the image, and keep your awareness focused on what you feel.
- Imagine that the part of you with no fear is offering comfort to the image of your suffering.
- Recognize that you don't need to change anything. You don't need to be "fixed." Practice simply accepting what is.
- You may offer yourself a silent blessing, such as "May you be free from suffering." Or you can simply sit with awareness, with an open heart, and without fear.
- When you're ready, let go of the image of yourself suffering. Bring to mind another person who is suffering in some way.
- Sit as long as you'd like with an openhearted awareness of the other person and a genuine desire to see his or her suffering relieved.

⟨⟫

FORGIVENESS

Practicing loving-kindness is hard. We often feel envy, or resentment, or bitterness, or even hatred—that's just the way it is. Or we harbor an unwillingness to forgive, even if we think we should. We can't expect ourselves to never have these thoughts or feelings. So rather than seek perfection, the solution to is to create a peaceful heart. And out of that peace, it is possible to wish another well.

This is not denial or wishful thinking. We all have painful experiences. We all know people who have hurt us or whom we have hurt. Sometimes, we are even the ones hurting ourselves. We don't need to deny any of this. In fact, it's crucial for us to tell the truth about it, to feel the painful feelings of which we've just become aware. But we don't want to get stuck with that pain, so we practice cultivating the heart, opening it, and letting go of what burdens it.

One of the most challenging aspects of a heartfulness practice is forgiveness. Intuitively, we know that holding on to bitterness or resentment only extends the harm of the original injury. We know that it's in our own best interest to forgive another, but somehow we just can't. Sometimes it seems to me that the more painful is the wound, the more tightly we hold on to it.

Sometimes when the notion of forgiveness is brought up, people say "He (or she) doesn't *deserve* to be forgiven." That may be so. But *you* deserve to have the capacity to forgive, whether you decide to grant this boon or not.

Some spiritual writers have suggested that we humans are not able to forgive, that we need God to open our hearts to the possibility of forgiveness or letting go. I personally wouldn't argue with that perspective. But even if the final step in forgiveness is divine intervention, we are the only ones who can create the inner conditions to welcome this intervention and permit the divine to do its work.

A Meditation on Forgiveness

- Sit quietly in a comfortable position.
- Focus upon several breaths, allowing your mind to settle.
- Bring your awareness to the person needing your forgiveness, whether that is yourself or another. Hold an image of this person in your awareness.
- Notice whatever feeling is in your body at this moment, and accept it just as it is. Recognize that you don't have to have "good" or "positive" feelings. Be honest with yourself and accept whatever is true for you right now.
- Turn your awareness to the center of your chest and invite your heart to open, even slightly. If you are unable to open your heart, don't worry. Just hold the intention to be openhearted.
- If you have not done so before, tell yourself the truth about what happened. Include both your part in the situation and the other's.

Note: If telling yourself what really happened is difficult for you, you may want to complete this step outside of the meditation, working with a person who is skilled at listening. Or you could write about what happened.

- Experience whatever emotions come up. Try to observe them with open curiosity without fanning the flames or holding on to your feelings. Just watch your emotions arise, hold them lightly with your observing awareness, and watch them change. Eventually, they will pass (although it may take many meditations before they do).
- When you're ready, invite yourself to release the negative emotions—anger, resentment, bitterness, hostility, hatred—whatever is there.
- If and when it feels right, you may offer the other a blessing. Try to make it an honest wishing well. "May you be free from suffering. May you be released from anger. May you be judged fairly. May you be forgiven." You needn't say anything that doesn't feel true for you. If you sincerely want the other person to be happy, you might wish, "May you be filled with joy and happiness." If "May you be judged fairly" is all you can manage, that's okay, too.
- Close with a moment of thanks to yourself that you are willing to engage in such a difficult but transforming practice.

LIVING WITH A FULL HEART

As with the mindfulness practice, you will find that you continually fall away from your heartfulness practice. Although you'd like to be loving, compassionate, generous, forgiving, you simply don't feel that way all the time. And as before, that's just not a problem. Every time you realize that your heart is not open or benevolent, you simply need to recognize that fact and try as best you can to return to a loving state. The practice is not "feeling love all the time." The practice is "becoming aware of the state of your heart, and continually returning to the highest, most loving state that you can imagine for yourself."

Miraculously, your idea of what is highest and what is possible will change. With every step toward wholeness and joyfulness, the possibilities expand further. You are enlarging your container, and there is no end to that process.

THE SOUL IS MEANT FOR JOY

It is Unity that doth enchant me. By her power I am
free . . . happy in sorrow, rich in poverty, and quick
even in death.

—GIORDANO BRUNO, *On the
Infinite Universe and Worlds*

One of the great enemies of joy is the misguided belief that we are
ultimately isolated beings. We believe that we are each a separate self
that needs to be protected, nurtured, and sustained. Yet it is the very nature of separation to make us unhappy and unfulfilled, so that we feel as
if we don't quite belong, as if the flow of life somehow passes around us
without touching us. These beliefs are continually reinforced in our culture, where nearly everyone shares them. But I would like to suggest to
you the possibility that this notion of the separate self is only an illusion, albeit a very powerful and well-supported one.

Our belief in separation is perhaps never quite so strong as when we
are in the midst of depression. Feeling alone, unworthy, and unloved at
such times adds further to our suffering. The more alone we feel, the
more we withdraw, in a vicious cycle that only reinforces the illusion
that got us unto trouble in the first place. "Why are you unhappy?" asks
the ancient Chinese sage. He answers: "Because nearly everything that
you say and do is for your 'self,' and there isn't one!"

This notion of human unity is a very difficult concept for those of us
who are embedded in Western culture. Much of the American story involves the rise of the individual, with a focus on individual rights and
responsibilities, accumulation and protection of private assets, and personal growth and self-actualization. So when philosophers talk about
"unity," we have trouble even understanding what they mean, much less
accepting it.

I'm not suggesting that you give up your appreciation for your individual self, a person with your own boundaries—and your own unique
gifts to share with the world. I'm only saying that until you also experience yourself as part of the whole, you'll never have a reliable access to
joy.

As Bruno observed in the quotation above, happiness is possible at any moment, even in the midst of sorrow. Joy is not the absence of suffering, nor the opposite of sadness. Joy is simply the natural outcome of *knowing* and *feeling* the connection that your soul longs for.

Though we are in fact always connected, most of the time we don't know it. We choose instead the illusion of separation, without even realizing that we're making a choice.

A TAPROOT TO JOY

Joy isn't an object or an achievement. It's more like a gentle breeze that simply comes, on its own, when it's allowed to do so. But if joy is really natural, why doesn't it come to us more often and more easily?

Usually, joy is not present because we haven't allowed it to be. We block it chemically, with unbalanced biochemicals in our brain, with poor nutrition that depletes our bodies, or sleep patterns that disrupt our relationship to nature and our own cycles. We block it with our thoughts, when we strive to control the uncontrollable, to grasp after happiness, to push away love and connection, to blind ourselves to internal and external reality. We block it with our hearts, too, when we close down in fear or resentment or confusion. You cannot receive an object when your hand is clenched. You cannot receive food when your jaws are clenched. You cannot receive joy when your mind is clenched. And you cannot receive love when your heart is clenched.

We also block joy when we refuse to become aware. People who aren't conscious don't realize what they have, don't feel the energies that flow continually in them and around them. They don't know that they reside in a sea of plenty. Unconscious people may experience moments of happiness, when one of their wants is satisfied. But such temporary satisfaction can never lead to lasting joy.

People who are blocked, closed, or unaware are like people whose only source of water is the rain. The rain comes when it will, allowing them to quench their thirst and find happiness for a while. But the rain can't fall forever, and eventually, thirst returns. If the rain stays away for weeks or months, then the earth dries, the crops wilt, and all the land is parched.

But people who are conscious don't need to depend on the rain, though they, too, may enjoy it when it comes. It's as though they've realized that the earth holds an unending supply of fresh water, just below the surface. Conscious, mindful people don't have to search frantically for water to satisfy their thirst. They simply tap into that reservoir and draw from it freely, using it lavishly and with abandon.

Of course no one is mindful and awake all the time. Even when you know the secret of the endless reservoir, you might find a way to block its flow into your heart and soul, or you might fail to maintain your connection to this underground source. But so long as you remain conscious, you will know that joy is there. You will understand that a blocked flow is by definition a temporary problem that simply needs to be addressed.

So if you want to achieve "enlightenment," wake up to this awareness that joy and love are all around you—but they're only accessible if we send our taproot down. Send it deep enough, and you can strike the reservoir and drink from it daily. Each of us has such a taproot living within us. This is what I would call the soul.

LISTENING TO YOUR SOUL

My sense is that the soul always wants to communicate. But we aren't very good at listening. Maybe our lives are too hectic or our minds too busy to take the time and patience to hear its "still, small voice." Perhaps we'd rather not hear what our soul has to say, fearful that we might have to change our lives in challenging ways, give up a prized attitude, take fearsome chances. Or maybe we simply don't recognize the importance of listening to the soul.

I believe that soul always wants what is best for us, even if we can't see that at the time. It will never lead us astray. Indeed, when we fall out of touch with our souls, we become troubled. Then the soul may be forced to emerge somehow, to make its presence known, to do whatever it must to slow us down, to give us pause, to help us to hear.

Sometimes, depression may stem from such a communication: "Stop! Slow down! Listen to your life! You have taken a wrong turn—change course now, before it is too late!" From this point of view, depression—despite or perhaps because it causes us to contract our lives and disengage from the world around us—can also serve as an opening.

To imagine this opening, I like to draw on theologian Marcus Borg's use of the Celtic concept of "thin places": the times in life when the situation we're in contrives to open us up so that the divine might enter. Particularly in times of hardship, we become more permeable than usual, more open to the forces of love and enlightenment or spirit. Depression can be such a thin place.

What can you do to be more open to the voice of the soul? First, I'd counsel you against rushing too quickly back to life as usual. After all, something about "life as usual" probably had a role in creating your depression. Of course I'm not suggesting that you remain depressed. But you may experience a time of tenderness, of vulnerability, that you'll notice if you listen carefully to your heart.

The early days of recovery are an excellent time to practice loving-kindness toward yourself, both in meditation and through action. It is also a time to let others practice kindness toward you. Allow friends to call upon you, to express their love and caring, to be generous toward you. Accept it gratefully. Often, others don't know how to respond to a person who's depressed. If you know such people, you might consider telling them what you'd like. Author and teacher Parker Palmer tells the story of a most helpful visitor who spoke little but who sat with Parker during his depression and rubbed his feet. The love embodied in that gesture, along with the connecting power of touch, did a great deal to keep Parker going through his darkest times.

Because you can be more open at this time, you may receive more wisdom than when you're caught up in business as usual. But mind your language, so that you don't berate, criticize, or diminish yourself in any way. The soul reveals itself only under the most inviting conditions.

So hold open the possibility that deep healing may come from your experience with depression—healing that you couldn't have accessed any other way. Mindfulness, heartfulness, and soulfulness can all help you heal. Perhaps this raw and tender time is softening you up for joy.

Depression can be a devastating experience, one that literally lays waste to the familiar landscape of our life. But in the silence that follows a destructive storm, we may be attuned to hear new sounds; and in the exhaustion that follows a bout with depression, we may finally be ready to listen. In such circumstances, one of the most healing things we can do for ourselves is to begin a dialogue with our soul.

SPEAKING WITH YOUR SOUL

Creating a relationship with your inner self—your soul or essence—is similar to developing any meaningful relationship. You meet, there is some degree of attraction, you spend time together, you talk, you listen, you respect each other. Over time, perhaps you grow very familiar and even come to love each other. Although many of us have had this experience with other humans, very few of us have established relationships with our souls. We may not realize that we need time to build this relationship, just like any other, or that we need the patience to allow the other to reveal itself in its own time, its own way.

Meditation is one way to reconnect with your soul. Prayer is another. But I also find it useful to speak directly with your essential self, through a technique I call "Dialogue with Your Inner Voice." Here's a description of how to begin such a dialogue.

Dialogue with Your Inner Voice

- Set aside enough time to establish a meaningful dialogue. You might commit to spending one hour a week for three months, or develop some other schedule that feels right. But having made the commitment, stick to it. Although your soul may be longing to speak to you, it may be more cautious than you expect. If you were trying to coax a wild animal out of the forest, you couldn't expect it to emerge on your first or even your fourth try. You would need to sit quietly at the edge of the woods, waiting for the relationship to take its own shape.

- Buy a special journal to use just for these dialogues. Keeping a separate notebook makes a statement to you—and to your soul—that you value it in a special way and that you intend to take these dialogues seriously.

- Find a quiet place to write free of interruptions. Just the process of committing to this separate, private time makes a powerful statement to your soul that you are ready to listen in a new way.

- Begin by quieting your mind. Close your eyes for a moment. Ask for guidance and request the presence of spirit during the time of your dialogue.

- Frame a question, a concern, or a dilemma on which you seek guidance. If you had access to the world's wisest sage, what would you ask? Find that question and prepare to ask it.

- Write the question in your journal. Then begin to wait. Sooner or later an idea, an image, or words will form in your mind. (Hint: The more relaxed you are about the arrival of this response, the sooner and more easily it will come. You know the expression "A watched pot never boils"? Well, an eagerly awaited "soul answer" may not "boil" either. Wait patiently—and not too avidly—for your soul to come to you.

- When you feel that something is coming to you, write it down, just as it comes. Don't censor, edit, analyze, or force the answer. Just write until it feels complete.
- When you've written what you've "heard," go on to write down your next contribution to the dialogue, either a response to the answer that has just come, or another question. Continue for as long as you have time, or until you feel finished. Then do your best to follow the guidance that you've received.
- Return to this practice as often as you would like, especially when faced with difficult decisions or stressful times.

Signs of Authenticity in a Soul Dialogue

- You feel a sense of clarity and a lack of ambiguity.
- Your soul's voice is completely benevolent, never harsh or critical.
- While the words or ideas you receive may challenge or redirect you, you hear no judgment, shaming, or blame.
- You respond with an internal resonance: You know Truth when you hear it.
- You feel a quickening, a bringing to life that comes through the words.
- You feel that the dialogue is moving you forward, guiding you toward a fuller, richer, more beautiful life.
- The voice you hear seems compassionate toward you and others. The words are filled with kindness and love.
- The dialogue draws you into relationship with others and helps you experience a deep connection with humanity—the sense of unity that Bruno identified.
- If you attend to your heart as you are writing or reading, you'll feel a sense of openness and a flowing of energy.
- After the dialogue, you'll feel lighter, less burdened, totally supported.
- If you ask for it, you will be given very specific guidance and suggestions.

CONNECTING WITH OTHERS:
THE CALL TO COMMUNITY

Civilization is a process in the service of Eros,
whose purpose is to combine single human
individuals, and after that families, then races,
peoples and nations, into one great unity, the unity
of mankind.

—SIGMUND FREUD,
Civilization and Its Discontents

Over the past hundred and fifty years, the West has seen a well-documented transformation from a society based on community to one based upon the individual. Whereas we once felt a moral obligation for one another's welfare, we now rely more upon law and contracts to determine how to treat one another. And instead of being connected by stories of meaning—religious teachings, mythic tales, political principles, or other ideals—we now draw our binding principles from science.

I believe our experience of depression, while having been eased in many ways by the focus on science, has also been made harder on that account. Of course depression has never been an easy or welcome experience. But it used to be viewed as an opportunity to come to terms with our lives in new ways. For example, the biblical psalms tell the story of King Saul finding comfort in David's music. Dante's *Inferno* recounts the tale of young Dante, "lost in a dark wood," descending to hell and struggling to find his own way out. The Christian mystics' "dark night of the soul" and the poetry of Rainer Maria Rilke are other examples of the richness that had been found in the experience we now call depression—richness that the sufferer then shared with the community.

Contrast that spiritual and communal perspective with our modern approach to depression, which we have come to see as an illness that can be medicated and treated with a few outcome-focused therapy sessions. The individual, facing a hell that we all might know, is nonetheless left essentially alone to deal with the crisis, which is understood in purely medical terms. In my view, this isolation only contributes to the depression; indeed, feeling disconnected may have partly caused the depression in the first place.

As much as anything, depression is a call to community, a stark reminder that we cannot go it alone—we are simply not designed that way. In the end, I believe, we need one another to heal, and the creation of community is just as important to our well-being as is the inner journey of coming to know ourselves.

Poet David Whyte has devised the expression "building a house of belonging," an effort he believes is central to the attempt of "making a home in the world." To build your own house of belonging, you need to start with a clear vision in your mind of the home you wish to inhabit. Here's an exercise to help you start developing that vision.

Building a House of Belonging

- Sit in a comfortable position.
- Close your eyes and take a few calming, mindful breaths.
- Bring to mind your own ability to create a loving community. Know that this creation is within your power if you focus your intention and take a few simple actions.
- Know that the belief that we are separate beings who must look out for ourselves is false. The deeper truth is that we are connected to one another and are here to care for one another.
- Direct your attention to your heart center. Allow for as much softening of the heart as you can. Invite an awareness of your deep longing for connection. Fully accept your own need for relationship and love.
- Bring to mind several meaningful people in your life, from now or from the past: loved ones, children, friends, colleagues, teachers, neighbors, mentors. See each person in his or her most loving form.
- Invite these beloved people, one at a time, to enter your heart center. Experience gratitude for what each one has meant to you. See yourself thanking them, embracing them. Release each image to bring up another. Repeat this process until you feel replete.
- See yourself as open and loving, part of a community of closeness and support. Envision yourself giving as much as receiving.
- End with a few moments of simply sitting, aware of your own heart and of your gratitude for all the loving people in your life.
- Repeat this practice daily, or as often as you like. You might consider adding someone new each time, either from your memory or from your daily experiences. Stay alert as you move through each day, seeking a new person whom you might add to this exercise.

CREATING CIRCLES OF TRUST

Although we're used to thinking of inner work as a journey we must take alone, I often feel that just the opposite is true. Often, we're best able to access our own inner wisdom when we're working in community, embedded within what Parker Palmer has called a "circle of trust" composed of like-minded souls. With a little effort and intention, we can create favorable conditions for the shy soul to appear and be heard in the presence of others.

༄

Building a Soul Community

- Abandon the notion that we know what is going on with the mystery of another—but don't abandon the other. Instead, firmly and gently hold a place for each of us to explore our own mystery.
- Believe that we all have the inner resources to find our own answers and solve our own problems.
- Don't try to "fix" others, or even see them as needing to be fixed. Refrain from offering advice, suggestions, or remedies.
- Don't judge or criticize, but rather listen with an open heart and acceptance.
- Honor silence. A still space is often the haven from which new insights or awareness can flow.
- Invite participation, but don't force it.
- Remain open to learning from one another.
- Value questions as much as answers and accept the wisdom in not knowing.

༄

SOUL FRIENDS

The Buddhist term *kalyanamitra* refers to "soul friends," companions who help one another along their spiritual paths. This concept is also one found in the Christian tradition, in which a person who's completed a spiritual journey serves as a mentor or friend to another who is embarking upon that journey. In both the Buddhist and the Christian tradition, deep listening is the cornerstone of these soul friendships.

We all need someone in our lives who really knows how to listen. When someone listens not with their ears or their thinking mind, but with an open heart and a nonjudging mind, then the soul feels safe to come out and reveal itself. The speaker has been empowered to go deeper into the story than before, to speak from the heart, uncensored and unfiltered. This kind of exchange is a gift for both the speaker and the listener, a relationship that goes beyond the unequal roles of helper and helped, therapist and client, healer and wounded one. Rather, the exchange is a relationship of two souls, in which "the god in me meets the god in you" and both parties are the richer for it. The remarkable thing about such a soul relationship is that whether you are the speaker or the listener, you benefit a great deal.

Deep listening depends more upon the presence of the listener than on his or her technique, upon *being* rather than *doing*. Most of us Westerners are conditioned to react, to take charge. We tend to forget that the best course of action is sometimes nonaction, as embodied in the twelve-step motto "Don't just do something—stand there!" Mindfulness helps train us to listen in this way—calm, detached, present, but not interfering or reacting, simply observing.

The thinking mind must be relatively quiet for you to engage in this kind of listening. If you're listening, you don't need to figure anything out or fix the other's problem. You don't even need to support, advise, or share a similar story from your own life. As you listen, you aren't thinking of what you'll say in response or when it's your turn to speak. Instead, you'll sidestep your own thoughts and simply be present.

At such times, I find it most helpful to turn to heart awareness, because for me this automatically quiets the mind. And when I am open to receiving another's story, I am invariably touched by it, and that opens the heart even further, making my listening more effective. You can be sure that if you feel moved by what a person is saying to you, they sense that and know that you are truly present with them. You don't need to say a thing, because this knowing is communicated without words.

In addition to presence, deeply listening requires time. Although the highly skilled listener can become fully present in just a moment, it takes time to create the context for deep listening, the sense of spaciousness required for the other to feel safe enough to truly open up.

Time, presence, nonjudging awareness, seeing the wholeness in another, listening to a story without needing to comfort or fix—these are the makings of a deep friendship. Learning to listen well, and finding someone willing and able to do that for you, are great ways to cultivate deep friendships.

Deep Listening Exercise

- Find another person whom you trust and who is willing to both speak and listen.
- Set aside thirty to forty-five minutes when you won't be interrupted.
- Take turns as speaker, allowing ten to fifteen minutes for each person.
- You may speak about any topic that is important to you, or just speak about your current experience. Examples of topics might include:
  - Describe when you are most alive and what brings you to life.
  - Recall a time when someone saw more in you than you saw in yourself. Describe the person, listing the qualities that allowed them to see so much in you and telling what effect their listening had upon you.
  - Discuss your experience with vocation. What were your first signs pointing you toward your life's work? What has influenced your career choices? Do you feel a sense of calling in what you do now? If so, how can you support that calling; if not, how might you get back to a sense of vocation?
  - Discuss a dilemma, a choice you have to make, a problem that you can't see through clearly and would like help in discerning.
- It doesn't matter too much what you choose. The important thing is that you choose a topic that has real meaning for you and that you have the experience of being deeply heard.
- When it's your turn to speak, speak from the heart. Don't think too much about what to say or how to say it. Don't censor your speech. Let go of any need to please the listener, impress, or entertain. Just speak what is true for you.
- When it's your turn to listen, just listen. Let the words fall upon you like raindrops, effortlessly. You don't need to strain to discern each one, or to think about a response. You don't even need to respond at all. If you feel like jumping in with a thought or a suggestion, restrain yourself. Stay with listening. If you say anything at all, it should only be to ask a clarifying question about which you genuinely wonder, not a prompt for which you think that you have an answer.

- Avoid the usual gestures by which we mark so much of our communication—the head nod, the smile, saying "uh-huh," or any other way of letting the person know you're listening. As speaker, try not to look for these signs. It may free you both if you don't even make eye contact during the exercise.
- If an emotion arises, just let it be. You might notice your urge to comfort or try to make things better. But feeling what is truly there may be just what your partner needs, far more than being consoled or advised. Notice, too, if you are uncomfortable with expressions of emotion. If your partner has entrusted you with his or her truth, just hold this awareness lightly and then return to listening. Your partner can take care of him or herself, finding great comfort in your quiet presence.
- Be comfortable with silence. Don't feel a need to fill it with speech, either as speaker or as listener. If the silence feels awkward, just sit with the awkwardness.
- Take care not to judge each other. Whenever a judgment arises, notice it and let it go. If you think you "see their problem" or know how to "fix it," let those thoughts go, too. The truth is, you don't know. Resist the temptation to offer "help."
- Allow for ample time for each person to speak. Know that you don't need to "get it all out" or come to any resolution. There will be opportunities to return to conversation it if it is truly important.

BEING DRAWN TOWARD PURPOSE

I believe that our highest purpose is determined by the soul, which enters this life with something "written on it." Our soul's purpose is not a blueprint, with all the instructions clearly spelled out, nor a mission statement, with specified goals and objectives. Our soul's purpose is more like a thread that runs through your life, gently pulling you toward your destiny. The thread is unbreakable, though it can become frayed, tangled, or unraveled, drawing you forward by inspiring you with longing for your deepest desires. You know you are following your soul's thread when you feel a sense of completeness, of deep satisfaction, or when the voice of longing becomes silent because you have that which you most truly desire.

But finding your own truth is not a once-and-for-all task. Your soul's purpose reveals itself a little at a time, a road "you make by walking." But even as you create your own new path, you still need specific landmarks or destination points to guide you along the way.

One such signpost is the point at which things become unnecessarily difficult. A certain amount of difficulty can be stimulating, even inspiring, but if you're not enjoying yourself, are experiencing undue stress, or are feeling bored or tired, that may be a message that you have lost the thread. Sometimes unhappiness is your best guide.

Another signpost is to notice what draws you. So often, we're motivated by what we think we should do, or by what we think others want or need from us. It's so much healthier to let yourself be drawn by that which holds a deep attraction to you, so long as your longing doesn't turn into grasping or need. If you let yourself be guided by what you most love, you'll have found a fairly accurate guide to your purpose.

⊙ﾑﾑﾑ⊙

Guided Imagery Exercise: Tending Your Inner Garden

- Sit in a comfortable position.
- Close your eyes and take a few calming, mindful breaths.
- Imagine yourself standing in a garden in the early spring, after the ground has thawed but before the plants have come up.
- Look around you and survey the landscape. See where you are drawn, then go there.
- Bend or kneel down and remove the debris from last fall and winter. What does that debris look and feel like? What does it symbolize in your life now?
- Now look and see the old, dead remnants that lie beneath the debris. Are there new shoots? What is the new life, waiting to come forth in your life? What needs to be cleared before they can emerge?
- See yourself cutting and pulling, raking and clearing the garden space.
- Look again at your garden. Is it overly crowded, or too sparse? If there are openings, what would you like to place there? If there is no room, what is most important to you, and what can you remove so that the important plants can thrive?

- Spend as much time as you would like with these images. Then allow fifteen to twenty minutes to write about what you observed.
- If possible, find a good listener to talk to about this experience.

RETURNING TO YOUR TRUE HOME

One of the most compelling images in the spiritual literature is that of one who has wandered in the desert but eventually finds the way home. In such stories, the desert can be seen as a metaphor for suffering, while home is a symbol of joy and belonging. Depression is surely a desert experience. But what is the home to which you return when the journey is over?

One of the great mysteries of depression is how such a desert experience, such a time of misery and loneliness, can leave you enlarged and deepened. Here are some signs of having successfully completed your journey through depression, some things that you may hope for on the other side:

- A body that is aligned and free of pain.
- A mind that is balanced and calm, free of fear and anxiety. A mind that serves you, but does not control you.
- A heart that is large and open and filled with love and kindness for all—including yourself. Your heart feels safe and secure, with no need to hide nor close itself off in protection.
- A soul that remains as healthy and resilient as it has ever been. By definition, your soul has always remained true to you. But now you are listening to it, being directed by it, abiding by it.

The chemistry of joy is based on aligning your body, mind, and heart in service to your soul and its design. Your soul will teach you how to be fully in this world and how to give yourself to that which you are meant to do. Choose to follow this path with all of yourself, wholeheartedly, and you will be a whole, vital, joyous human being.

Perfection is a deadly, impossible goal, and seeking it will bring us only frustration. What we need to seek instead is fuller growth into who we really are, the possibility of being here now. Sometimes this quest for being will bring you joy, serenity, even a kind of triumph as you feel yourself overcoming old blocks and reconnecting to your true potential. Sometimes the same quest brings further lessons to learn, an illness or misalignment that needs healing, or the need to be loved or cared for by another. This is a never-ending journey, for there is always more that you can be. Joy is available to you at every step, not as a goal that you are moving toward, but as a pleasing companion along the journey.

Declare this desert experience to be over. Accept yourself and your experience, and in that very acceptance of where you are, become ready to move on. Be willing to be reanimated with energy and purpose, to allow your heart to reawaken and reopen. Be willing to let spirit reenter your life, guiding your next steps in the journey. Allow yourself to become a crucible for the chemistry of joy.

APPENDIX A

Serotonin-Enhancing Foods

High-tryptophan Protein
Turkey
Milk, cheese, cottage cheese
Eggs

Whole Grains
Brown rice
Quinoa
Oatmeal
Whole-grain breads and pastas

Beans and Legumes
Soybeans (try edamame, fresh green soybeans)
Black beans
Fava beans
Pinto beans
Chickpeas
Kidney beans
Lima beans
Split peas
Lentils

Root Vegetables
Carrots
Beets
Potatoes
Sweet potatoes
Onions
Turnips
Rutabagas
plus Squash and Pumpkins

Nuts *(daily serving size in parentheses)*
Almonds (10 to 15)
Walnuts (6 to 10)
Pecans (10 to 15 halves)
Pistachios (20 to 30)
Cashews (6 to 10)
Peanuts (20 to 30) or peanut butter (1 to 2 tablespoons)

Seeds *(1 to 3 tablespoons per day)*
Pumpkin
Sunflower
Sesame
Flaxseeds

Green, Yellow, Red, and Leafy Vegetables
These foods don't contain any tryptophan themselves, but they are terrific sources of the B vitamins and minerals that the brain needs to turn tryptophan into serotonin. They're also are great sources of fiber, antioxidants, and cancer-preventing agents.

Garlic
If you want to get the most benefit from garlic, eat it raw, or else crush it and leave it to sit for fifteen minutes before cooking.

Dopamine/Norepinephrine—Enhancing Foods

Lean Beef
Sirloin steak (with the fat cut off) or ground low-fat sirloin
Top round or flank steak
Tenderloin (with the fat trimmed off)

Lean Pork
Low-fat ham
Canadian bacon
Tenderloin

Turkey
Fat-free sliced turkey
Turkey breast
Low-fat turkey bacon or sausage

Chicken
Fat-free sliced chicken
Chicken breast—grilled, broiled, or stir-fried
Low-fat chicken sausage

Seafood
Cold-water fish—salmon, mackerel, herring, or sardines—which are especially good for Omega-3 fatty acids.
Note: Recent news reports have raised some concern about farm-raised salmon having too many contaminants. Until salmon farmers improve their practices, look for wild Alaskan salmon—*Atlantic* is often a code word for "farmed."

Other fish, including tuna, halibut, and cod. They don't have as many Omega-3s but are excellent low-fat protein sources.
Shrimp and other shellfish and crustaceans

Other Meats
Wild game, like deer or pheasant—they can be lean and also good sources of Omega-3s
Bison—it tastes different from beef, and is lean and healthy
Ostrich—also a very lean meat

Dairy Products
Fat-free cottage cheese. This is pure protein, and a good thing to mix with fruit or salad. About a half cup makes a full serving of protein.
Cheese. Low-fat cheeses such as part-skim mozzarella or string cheese are also mostly protein with very little fat. Hard cheeses have protein, too, and are great sources of flavor, though they do include more fat.
Yogurt. You can enjoy a cup of low-fat or nonfat yogurt without added sugar or sweetened fruit for a very balanced source of protein and carbohydrate.
Milk. Because milk itself has a much higher percentage of carbohydrate than other dairy products, I wouldn't consider it a serving of protein, but it

does offer you some protein along with calcium and, if you're drinking enriched milk, vitamin D.

Other Protein Sources

Eggs: This healthy all-around food offers you a high-quality protein source. Yolks do have a lot of arachidonic acid, a substance that contributes to inflammation, so if you've got an inflammatory condition—including autoimmune conditions, asthma, arthritis, and certain skin conditions—you might want to avoid or reduce your intake of egg yolks. Most of us, though, can feel free to enjoy eggs—complete with yolks—from pasture-raised, flax-fed hens. I'd avoid the mass-produced eggs that are high in Omega-6s and probably loaded with toxins as well.

Tofu: Look for low-fat or light tofu if you can, and of course, avoid deep-frying.

Protein powders: These are quick and easy to use, especially at breakfast time, and they make it easy for vegetarians to ensure that they are getting enough protein. I recommend soy protein powder; nonsoy vegetable protein powder; rice protein powder; whey powder; and egg powder, which is made from egg whites only.

Beans and Legumes

Soy beans (try edamame, or fresh green soybeans)
Black beans
Fava beans
Pinto beans
Chickpeas
Kidney beans
Lima beans
Split peas
Lentils
Peanuts (20 to 30) or peanut butter (1 to 2 teaspoons)

Nuts *(daily serving size in parentheses)*
Almonds (10 to 15)
Walnuts (6 to 10)
Pecans (10 to 15 halves)
Pistachios (20 to 30)
Cashews (6 to 10)

Seeds *(1 to 3 tablespoons per day)*
Pumpkin
Sunflower
Sesame
Flaxseeds

Green, yellow, red, and leafy vegetables

These are not themselves sources of norepi/dopa, but of the B vitamins and minerals that are essential to the brain in making this vital neurotransmitter. And of course, brightly colored veggies are great sources of fiber, antioxidants, and cancer-preventing agents.

APPENDIX C

Resources

**Alternative Medicine
Practitioners:**
American Academy of
Environmental Medicine
7701 East Kellogg, Suite 625
Wichita, KS 67207
316-684-5500
www.aaem.com

American Association of
Naturopathic Physicians
3201 New Mexico Ave. NW,
Suite 350
Washington, DC 20016
866-538-2267
www.naturopathic.org

American College for Advancement
in Medicine
23121 Verdugo Dr., Suite 204
Laguna Hills, CA 92653
800-532-3688
www.acam.org

American Holistic Medical
Association
12101 Menaul Blvd. NE, Suite C
Albuquerque, NM 87112
505-292-7788
www.holisticmedicine.org

International Society for
Orthomolecular Medicine
www.orthomed.org

National Ayurvedic Medical
Association
620 Cabrillo Ave.
Santa Cruz, CA 95065
www.ayurveda-nama.org

Information and Education:
American Botanical Council
6200 Manor Rd.
Austin, TX 78723
512-926-4900
www.herbalgram.org

Center for Mindfulness in Medicine,
Health Care and Society
University of Massachusetts Medical
School
Worcester, MA 01655
www.umassmed.edu/cfm/

Center for Spirituality and Healing
University of Minnesota
Online and classroom courses,
research, events, and education
612-624-9459
www.csh.umn.edu

ConsumerLab.com
Independent laboratory testing on
herbs and supplements
www.consumerlab.com

Dr. Andrew Weil's Self Healing
Newsletter
www.drweilselfhealing.com

Herb Research Foundation
4140 15th St.
Boulder, CO 80304
303-449-2265
www.herbs.org

Medline
National Library of Medicine's search service
www.ncbi.nlm.nih.gov

Nutrition Action Healthletter
www.cspinet.org

Laboratories for Nutrient Level and Food Sensitivity Testing:
Great Smokies Diagnostic Laboratory
800-522-4762
www.greatsmokies-lab.com

Immuno Laboratories
800-231-9197
www.immunolabs.com

Pantox Laboratories
619-272-3885
www.pantox.com

Nutritional Supplements:
Advanced Physicians Products
800-220-7687
www.nutritiononline.com

Bioforce
877-232-6060
www.bioforce.com

Ethical Nutrients
800-668-8743
www.ethicalnutrients.com

Frontier Herbs
800-669-3275
www.frontiercoop.com

InVite
(multivitamin formulated by Dr. Andrew Weil)
800-203-0439
www.invitehealth.com

Nature Made
(good source for SAMe)
800-276-2878
www.naturemade.com

Nature's Way
(Maker of Perika, a reliable St. John's wort product)
801-489-1500
www.naturesway.com

Nordic Naturals
(good source for fish oil)
800-662-2544
www.nordicnaturals.com

Omegabrite
(good source of Omega-3 products)
800-383-2030
www.omegabrite.com

Rainbow Light
Multivitamins and antioxidants
800-635-1233
www.rainbowlight.com

Light Therapy Products:
Northern Light Technologies
800-263-0066
www.northernlighttechnologies.com

Physician Engineered Products
(800) 622-6240
www.feelbrightlight.com

Ayurvedic Resources:
Auromere, Inc.
800-735-4691
www.auromere.com

The Chopra Center
2013 Costa del Mar Rd.
Carlsbad, CA 92009
888-424-6772
www.chopra.com

Herbalvedic Products
262-889-8569
www.herbalvedic.com

Lotus Brands
800-889-8561
www.lotusbrands.com

Maharishi Ayurveda Products
800-255-8332
www.mapi.com

**Mindfulness Meditation Tapes
and Instruction:**
Insight Meditation Society
978-355-4378
www.dharma.org

Spirit Rock Meditation Center
415-488-0164
www.spiritrock.org

Sounds True
800-333-9185
www.soundstrue.com

Stress Reduction Tapes
(Tapes by Jon Kabat-Zinn)
P.O. Box 547
Lexington, MA 02420
www.stressreductiontapes.com
Or *www.mindfulnesstapes.com*

For meditation tapes or information
about workshops by Dr. Emmons, contact him at *www.henryemmonsmd.com*

NOTES

Chapter 4

1. E. M. Blass, E. Fitzgerald, and P. Kehoe, "Interactions between Sucrose, Pain and Isolation Distress." *Pharmacology, Biochemistry and Behavior* 26 (1986): 483–489.
2. K. DesMaisons, *Potatoes Not Prozac*. New York: Simon & Schuster, 1998.
3. P. F. Sullivan, et al., "Total Cholesterol and Suicidality in Depression." *Biological Psychiatry* 36 (1994): 472–477.
4. P. Godfrey, B. Toone, M. Carney, et al., "Enhancement of Recovery from Psychiatric Illness by Methylfolate." *Lancet* 336 (1990): 392–395.
5. I. Bell, J. Edman, F. Morrow, et al., "B Complex Vitamin Patterns in Geriatric and Young Adult Inpatients with Major Depression." *Journal of the American Geriatrics Society* 39 (1991): 252–257.
6. B. W. Penninx, J. M. Guralnik, et al., "Vitamin B_{12} Deficiency and Depression in Physically Disabled Older Women: Epidemiologic Evidence from the Women's Health and Aging Study." *American Journal of Psychiatry* 157 (May 2000): 715–721.
7. B. J. Kaplan, et al., "Effective Mood Stabilization with a Chelated Mineral Supplement: An Open-Label Trial in Bipolar Disorder." *Journal of Clinical Psychiatry* 62 (2001): 936–944; A. B. Mayer, "Historical Changes in the Mineral Content of Fruits and Vegetables." *British Food Journal*. 99 (1997): 207–211; C. W. Popper, "Do Vitamins or Minerals (Apart from Lithium) Have Mood-Stabilizing Effects?" *Journal of Clinical Psychiatry* 62, no. 12 (2001): 933–944; S. J. Schoenthaler and I. D. Bier, "The Effect of Vitamin-Mineral Supplementation on Juvenile Delinquency Among American Schoolchildren: A Randomized, Double-Blind Placebo-Controlled Trial." *Journal of Alternative and Complementary Medicine* 6 (February 2000): 7–17.
8. S. T. Marcolina, "Food for Thought: Organic." *Alternative Medicine Alert* 6, no. 7 (2003): 73–78; National Research Council, *Pesticides in the Diets of Infants and Children*. Washington, DC: National Academy Press, 1993; U.S. Environmental Protection Agency, "Pesticides." available at www.epa.gov/pesticides; Environmental Working Group, "Foods You'll Want to Buy Organic." available at www.foodnews.org/highpesticidefoods.php; V. Klinkenborg, "A Farming Revolution: Sustainable Agriculture." *National Geographic*, December 1995; 60–89; A. B. Mayer, "Historical Changes in the Mineral

Content of Fruits and Vegetables." *British Food Journal* 99 (1997): 207–211; P. Mader, et al., "Soil Fertility and Biodiversity in Organic Farming." *Science* 296 (2002): 1694–1697; K. Woese, et al., "A Comparison of Organically and Conventionally Grown Foods: Results of a Review of the Relevant Literature." *Journal of Food and Agriculture* 74 (1995): 281–293; V. Worthington, "Nutritional Quality of Organic Versus Conventional Fruits, Vegetables and Grains." *Journal of Alternative Complementary Medicine* 2 (April 2001): 161–173.

Chapter 5

1. I. Bell, J. Edman, F. Morrow, et al., "Brief Communication: Vitamin B_1, B_2 and B_6 Augmentation of Tricyclic Antidepressant Treatment in Geriatric Depression with Cognitive Dysfunction." *Journal of the American College of Nutrition* 11 (1992): 159–163.

2. P. Godfrey, B. Toone, M. Carney, et al., "Enhancement of Recovery from Psychiatric Illness by Methylfolate." *Lancet* 336 (1990): 392–395.

3. T. T. Baldewicz, K. Goodkin, et al., "Cobalamin Level Is Related to Self-Reported and Clinically-Rated Mood and to Syndromal Depression in Bereaved HIV-1+ and HIV-1- Homosexual Men." *Journal of Psychosomatic Research* 48, no. 2, (2000): 177–185.

4. B. W. Penninx, J. M. Guralnik, et al., "Vitamin B_{12} Deficiency and Depression in Physically Disabled Older Women: Epidemiologic Evidence from the Women's Health and Aging Study." *American Journal of Psychiatry* 157 (May 2000): 715–721.

5. J. Hintikka, T. Tolmunen, et al., "High Vitamin B_{12} Level and Good Treatment Outcome May Be Associated in Major Depressive Disorder." *BMC Psychiatry.* 3 (December 2, 2003): 17.

6. J. McBride, "Can Foods Forestall Aging?" *Agricultural Research.* 47, no. 2 (February 1999): 15–17.

7. D. Benton and R. Cook, "The Impact of Selenium Supplementation on Mood." *Biological Psychiatry* 29 (1991): 1092–1098.

8. C. W. Popper, "Do Vitamins or Minerals (Apart from Lithium) Have Mood-Stabilizing Effects?" *Journal of Clinical Psychiatry* 62, no. 12 (2001): 933–944.

9. See for example, A. Tanskanen, J. R. Hibbeln, J. Tuomilehto, et al., "Fish Consumption and Depressive Symptoms in the General Population in Finland." *Psychiatric Services* 52, no. 4 (2001): 529–531.

10. A. P. Simopoulos, "Overview of Evolutionary Aspects of Omega-3 Fatty Acids in the Diet." *World Review of Nutrition and Dietetics* 83 (1998): 1–11.

11. L. A. Horrocks and Y. K. Yeo, "Health Benefits of Docosahexaenoic Acid (DHA)." *Pharmacological Research* 40, no. 3 (1999): 211–225.

12. T. Hamazaki, et al., "The Effect of Docosahexaenoic Acid on Aggression in

Young Adults: A Placebo-Controlled Double-Blind Study." *Journal of Clinical Investigation* 97 (1996): 1129–1133.

13. K. S. Vaddadi, P. Courtney, et al., "A Double-Blind Trial of Essential Fatty Acid Supplementation In Patients with Tardive Dyskinesia." *Psychiatry Research* 27 (3) (1989): 313–323.

14. A. L. Stoll, et al., "Omega-3 Fatty Acids in Bipolar Disorder: A Preliminary Double-Blind, Placebo-Controlled Trial." *Archives of General Psychiatry* 56 (May 1999): 407–412.

15. M. Maes, A. Christophe, J. Delanghe, et al., "Lowered Omega-3 Polyunsaturated Fatty Acids in Serum Phospholipids and Cholesteryl Esters of Depressed Patients." *Psychiatry Research* 85 (1999): 275–291.

16. M. Maes and R. S. Smith, "Fatty Acids, Cytokines and Major Depression." *Biological Psychiatry* 43, no. 5 (1998): 313–314.

17. J. R. Hibbeln, et al., "Essential Fatty Acids Predict Metabolites of Serotonin and Dopamine in Cerebrospinal Fluid Among Healthy Control Subjects, and Early- and Late-Onset Alcoholics." *Biological Psychiatry* 44 (1998): 235–242.

18. W. F. Byerly, et al., "5-HTP: A Review of Its Antidepressant Efficacy and Adverse Effects." *Journal of Clinical Psychopharmacology* 7 (1987): 127–137.

19. L. J. Van Hiele, "1-5-HTP in Depression: The First Substitution Therapy in Psychiatry?" *Neuropsychobiology* 6 (1980): 230–240.

20. W. Poldinger, et al., "A Functional-Dimensional Approach to Depression: Serotonin Deficiency as a Target Syndrome in a Comparison of 5-HTP and Fluvoxamine." *Psychopathology* 24 (1991): 53–81.

21. H. M. van Praag and S. de Haan, "Depression Vulnerability and 5-Hydroxytryptophan Prophylaxis." *Psychiatry Research* 3 (1980): 75–83; H. M. van Praag, "In Search of the Mode of Action of Antidepressants: 5-HTP/Tyrosine Mixtures in Depression." *Advances in Biochemical Psychopharmacology* 39 (1984): 301–314; H. M. van Praag and R. S. Kahn, "L-5-Hydroxytryptophan in Depression and Anxiety." *Schweizerische Rundschau fur Medizin Praxis* 77, no. 34A (1998): 40–46.

22. H. Sabelli, "Amino Acid Precursors for Depression." *Psychiatric Times* (October 2000): 42–49; H. C. Sabelli and A. D. Mosnaim, "Phenylethylamine Hypothesis of Affective Behavior." *American Journal of Psychiatry* 131, no. 6 (1974): 695–699; H. C. Sabelli, et al., "Sustained Antidepressant Effect of PEA Replacement." *Journal of Neuropsychiatry Clinical Neurosciences* 8, no. 2 (1996): 168–171; W. Birkmayer, et al., "L-Deprenyl Plus L-Phenylalanine in the Treatment of Depression." *Journal of Neural Transmission* 59, no. 1 (1984): 81–87. H. C. Sabelli, "Phenylethylamine Replacement as a Rapid and Physiological Treatment for Depression." *Psycheline* 2, no. 3 (1998): 32–39.

23. D. B. Menkes, D. C. Coates, and J. P. Fawcett, "Acute Tryptophan Depletion Aggravates Premenstrual Syndrome." *Journal of Affective Disorders* 329, no. 1 (1994): 37–44.

24. "S-Adenyl-L-Methionine for Treatment of Depression, Osteoarthritis, and Liver Disease." *Evidence Report/Technology Assessment* 64 (October 2002): 1–194; R. P. Brown, P. Gerbarg, and T. Bottiglieri, "S-Adenylmethionine (SAMe) for Depression." *Psychiatric Annals* 32, no. 1 (2002): 29–44.

25. K. M. Bell, L. Plon, et al., "S-adenosylmethionine Treatment of Depression: A Controlled Clinical Trial." *American Journal of Psychiatry* 145, no. 9 (1988): 1110–1114.

26. R. P. Brown, P. Gerbarg, and T. Bottiglieri, "S-adenylmethionine (SAMe) for Depression." *Psychiatric Annals* 32, no. 1 (2002): 29–44.

27. J. Lake, "Psychotropic Medications from Natural Products: A Review of Promising Research and Recommendations." *Alternative Therapies* 6, no. 3 (2000): 36–60; B. Gaster and J. Holroyd, "St. John's Wort for Depression: A Systematic Review." *Archives of Internal Medicine* 160 (January 24, 2000): 152–156; E. Shrader, "Equivalence of St. John's Wort Extract and Fluoxetine: A Randomized, Controlled Study in Mild-Moderate Depression." *International Clinical Psychopharmacology* 15, no. 2 (2000): 61–68; L. Taylor and K. A. Kobak, "An Open-Label Trial of St. John's Wort in Obsessive Compulsive Disorder." *Journal of Clinical Psychiatry* 61 (August 2000): 575–578; J. R. T. Davidson and K. M. Connor, "St. John's Wort in Generalized Anxiety Disorder: Three Case Reports." *Journal of Clinical Psychopharmacology* 21 (2001): 635–636.

28. E.-P. Barrette, "St. John's Wort for the Treatment of Depression: An Update." *Alternative Medicine Alert* 6, no. 3 (2003): 25–30; U. Werneke, O. Horn, and D. M. Taylor. "How Effective is St. John's Wort? The Evidence Revisited." *Journal of Clinical Psychiatry* 65, no. 5 (May 2004): 611–617.

29. R. C. Shelton, M. B. Keller, et al., "Effectiveness of St. John's Wort in Major Depression: A Randomized Controlled Trial." *Journal of the American Medical Association* 285 (April 18, 2001): 1978–1986; Hypericum Depression Trial Study Group, "Effect of *Hypericum perforatum* (St. John's Wort) in Major Depressive Disorder: A Randomized Controlled Trial." *Journal of the American Medical Association* 287 (April 10, 2002): 1807–1814.

30. B. J. Diamond and S. C. Shiflett, "Ginkgo Biloba Extract: Mechanisms and Clinical Indications." *Archives of Physical Medicine and Rehabilitation* 81 (May 2000): 668–678; A. Fugh-Berman, *Alternative Medicine: What Works*. Tucson, Ariz.: Odonian Press, 1996, pp. 114–116; J. Lake, "Psychotropic Medications from Natural Products: A Review of Promising Research and Recommendations." *Alternative Therapies* 6, no. 3 (2000): 36–60.

31. P. L. Le Bars, M. M. Katz, et al., "A Placebo-Controlled, Double-Blind, Ran-

domized Trial of an Extract of *Ginkgo biloba* for Dementia." *Journal of the American Medical Association* 278 (1997): 1327–1332.

32. P. Le Bars, et al., "A 26-Week Analysis of a Double-Blind, Placebo-Controlled Trial of the Ginkgo Biloba Extract EGb 761 in Dementia." *Dementia and Geriatric Cognitive Disorders* 11, no. 4 (2000): 230–237.

33. A. J. Cohen and B. Bartlik, "Ginkgo Biloba for Antidepressant-Induced Sexual Dysfunction." *Journal of Sex and Marital Therapy* 24, no. 2 (1998): 139–144.

Chapter 6

1. J. Greist, M. Klein, et al., "Antidepressant Running: Running as Treatment for Nonpsychotic Depression." *Behavioral Medicine* 5 (1978): 19–24.

2. I. L. McCann and D. S. Holmes, "Influence of Aerobic Exercise on Depression." *Journal of Personality and Social Psychology* 46, no. 5 (1984): 1142–1147.

3. J. A. Blumenthal, M. A. Babyak, K. A. Moore, et al., "Effects of Exercise Training on Older Adults with Major Depression." *Archives of Internal Medicine* 159 (1999): 2349–2356.

4. M. Babyak, J. A. Blumenthal, S. Herman, et al., "Exercise Treatment for Major Depression: Maintenance of Therapeutic Benefit at Ten Months." *Psychosomatic Medicine* 62 (2000): 633–638.

5. Based on recommendations from the Centers for Disease Control and Prevention, the American College of Sports Medicine, and the Institute of Medicine.

6. A. C. King and R. F. Oman, et al., "Moderate-Intensity Exercise and Self-Rated Quality of Sleep in Older Adults. A Randomized Controlled Trial." *Journal of the American Medical Association* 277 (1997): 32–37.

7. D. Brown, "Valerian Root: Nonaddictive Alternative for Insomnia and Anxiety." *Review of Natural Medicine* (Fall 1994): 221–224.

8. F. Donath, S. Quispe, et al., "Critical Evaluation of the Effect of Valerian Extract on Sleep Structure and Sleep Quality." *Pharmacopsychiatry* 33 (2000): 47–53.

ACKNOWLEDGMENTS

It is with a deep sense of gratitude that I thank some of the many people who have helped to create this book. I start with my literary team: Janis Vallely, my agent, who called me with an idea for a book and who has shepherded this process with calm grace and firm patience. Nancy Hancock, the talented editor at Simon & Schuster, who took on this project with a degree of energy, commitment, and intelligence that I had only remotely hoped to find. Alison Rose Levy, a gifted writer with a passion for this subject, who helped with some of the early writing. And a very special thanks to Rachel Kranz. Our collaboration has been a natural and joyful one. Her energy, enthusiasm, and humor infuse this book with a life that I could not have given it alone. I am grateful for the end result, but also for the delightful process.

I thank the generous readers of my early manuscript, Jan Swanson, Sue Towey, and Sandy Kosse. All are friends and colleagues who not only read and revised, but helped shape the ideas in this book through our many years of working together. And I owe a great debt to Lisa DeLeon, whose reading and comments were done with a degree of care and competence that surprised and renewed me at just the right time.

I feel most fortunate to have had so many gifted colleagues, fellow teachers, and healers. Thanks to my partners in mindfulness teaching, Maggie Kessel, Dave Von Weiss, Joe Nelson, Julie Rice, Terry Pearson, and especially to my dharma sister, Kaia Svien, who brings a degree of love and compassion to her work that continually astounds me. Also, thanks to the many wonderful psychotherapists with whom I have had the good fortune to work, including my friends Susan Bourgerie and Sandy Kosse at the Loring Mindfulness Therapy Center. I am also surrounded by a community of healers, and I thank Hilmar Wagner, Jan Swanson, Jennifer Blair, Carolyn Denton, Bob Decker, Bohdan Melnychenko, Jeff Richards, Davis Taylor, and Gary Carlson for their unfailing support and encouragement. And a most gracious thanks to Mary Jo Kreitzer, Karen Lawson, and all the staff of the Center for Spirituality and Healing at the University of Minnesota, where I have been given so many opportunities to teach, learn, and share the lessons included in this book. I am particularly grateful to the Inner Life of Healers team, including Cass McLaughlin, Beth Somerville, and my wonderful teaching friends, Mary Catherine Casey and Laura Kinkead, with whom I learn and enjoy so much. I also wish to thank Andrea

Nelson and Beverly Pierce, Horst Rechelbacher, Bill and Penny George, and the Fetzer Foundation for helping to get that program off the ground.

I have had many exceptional teachers over the years who cannot know the impact they have had on me in the shaping of my mind and heart. Deepak Chopra and David Simon provided a sound background in Ayurvedic and Mind-Body medicine. James Gordon taught mind-body skills groups with great skill and passion. Jon Kabat-Zinn ignited my love of mindfulness meditation and changed the course of my career, as indeed he has changed the course of American medicine. His clarity, strength, and resolve continue to be an inspiration to me. Parker Palmer has taught me so much about the inner life and has done so with a humility and grace that makes him all the more loveable. His skill with the craft of writing and speaking about things that matter most deeply serve as a model that I could only hope to replicate. More than a mentor, I gladly count Parker and his wife, Sharon, among my friends. And Joe Bailey, who was first a teacher, then a colleague, and now like a brother. I thank both Joe and his wife, Michael, for their constant love and friendship.

I also want to acknowledge, with great tenderness and appreciation, the blessings that I have received from my patients. I have encountered thousands of souls, in varying degrees of suffering, who have entrusted to me some part of their lives and have enlarged my life in the process. Whatever benefits they have received from our work together, I have gotten back many times over. I thank them for partnering with me in the constant search for wholeness, which I understand as a never-ending movement toward love.

And finally, a warm embrace to my family: my wife, Jane, for her unwavering encouragement and support, and to our boys, Eric and Mark, who have been most gracious and patient to me in this entire process. They are, quite simply, my most constant source of love and joy.

INDEX

ABOUT THE AUTHOR

HENRY EMMONS, MD, is a psychiatrist who uses mind-body and alternative therapies in his clinical work. He has conducted workshops and retreats for health-care professionals on psychopharmacology, natural therapies for depression, the use of mindfulness meditation and health realization in medicine, resilience training, and the evolution from clinician to healer. Dr. Emmons has received training in Mindfulness Based Stress Reduction from Dr. Jon Kabat-Zinn and completed a Bush fellowship studying the integration of natural and alternative therapies in psychiatry. He has codeveloped and facilitated "A Year of Living Mindfully" and "The Inner Life of Healers" programs through the University of Minnesota's Center for Spirituality and Healing. He practices general and holistic psychiatry and consults to several colleges and organizations in and around Minneapolis–St. Paul.

ABOUT THE WRITER

RACHEL KRANZ has written numerous books on science, health, and psychology. She is the author of a novel, *Leaps of Faith*, and lives in New York City.